PLENTY

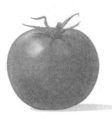

ONE MAN, ONE WOMAN, AND A
RAUCOUS YEAR OF EATING LOCALLY

PLENTY

ALISA SMITH AND J.B. MACKINNON

HARMONY BOOKS
NEW YORK

Published in the United States by Harmony Books, an imprint of the
Crown Publishing Group, a division of Random House, Inc., New York.
www.crownpublishing.com

Harmony Books is a registered trademark and the Harmony Books colophon
is a trademark of Random House, Inc.

Originally published in Canada in 2007 by Random House of Canada, Toronto.

Library of Congress Cataloging-in-Publication Data

Smith, Alisa, 1971–
    Plenty : one man, one woman, and a raucous year of eating locally / Alisa Smith
and J.B. MacKinnon.
        p.   cm.
    1. Diet—British Columbia. 2. Cookery (Natural foods)—British Columbia.
3. Farm produce—British Columbia. 4. Smith, Alisa, 1971– 5. MacKinnon, J.B.
(James Bernard), 1970– I. MacKinnon, J.B. (James Bernard), 1970– II. Title.
    TX360C32 B78 2007
    641.5'6309711—dc22   2006101586

ISBN 978-0-307-34732-9

Printed in the United States of America

10 9 8 7 6 5 4 3 2 1

First United States Edition

To maverick farmers, fishermen, gardeners, foragers,
and others feeding the future.

PLENTY

→❋ HERB TEA ❋←

1 LEAF SAGE

1 LEAF MINT

HOT WATER

PLACE THE FRESH-PICKED LEAVES IN A MUG. ADD WATER AT A ROLLING BOIL. STEEP FOR 6 MINUTES. A SIMPLE BEGINNING.

MARCH

The year of eating locally began with one beautiful meal and one ugly statistic.

First, the meal. What we had on hand, really, was a head of cabbage. Deep inside its brainwork of folds it was probably nourishing enough, but the outer layers were greasy with rot, as though the vegetable were trying to be a metaphor for something. We had company to feed, and a three-week-old cabbage to offer them.

It wasn't as though we could step out to the local megamart. We—Alisa and I—were at our "cottage" in northern British Columbia, more honestly a drafty, jauntily leaning, eighty-year-old homestead that squats in a clearing between Sitka spruce and western redcedar trees large enough to crush it into splinters with the sweep of a limb. The front door looks out on a jumble of mountains named after long-forgotten British lords, from the peaks of which you can see, just to the northwest, the southern

1

tip of the Alaska Panhandle. There is no corner store here. In fact, there is no electricity, no flush toilet, and no running water but for the Skeena River rapids known as the Devil's Elbow. They're just outside the back door. Our nearest neighbor is a black bear. There are also no roads. In fact, the only ways in or out are by canoe, by foot over the distance of a half-marathon to the nearest highway, or by the passenger train that passes once or twice a day, and not at all on Tuesdays. So: we had a cabbage, and a half-dozen mouths to feed for one more autumn evening. Necessity, as they say, can be a mother.

I can't remember now who said what, or how we made the plan, or even if we planned it at all. What I know is that my brother David, a strict vegetarian, hiked to the mouth of Fiddler Creek, which straight-lines out of a bowl of mountains so ancient they make you feel perpetually reborn, and reeled in an enormous Dolly Varden char. Our friends Kirk and Chandra, who are the sort of people who can tell a Bewick's wren from a rufous-crowned sparrow by ear, led a party into the forest and returned with pound upon pound of chanterelle, pine, and hedgehog mushrooms. I rooted through the tall grass to find the neglected garden plot where, months earlier, we had planted garlic and three kinds of potato; each turned up under the spade, as cool and autonomous as teenagers. Alisa cut baby dandelion leaves, while her mother picked apples and sour cherries from an abandoned orchard, and rose hips from the bushes that were attempting to swallow the outhouse. The fruit we steeped in red wine—all right, the wine came from Australia. Everything else we fried on the woodstove, all in a single huge pan.

It was delicious. It was a dinner that transcended the delicate freshness of the fish, the earthy goodness of the spuds that had sopped up the juices of mushrooms and garlic. The rich flavors were the evening's shallowest pleasure. We knew, now, that out there in the falling darkness the river and the forest spoke a subtle language we had only begun to learn. It was the kind of meal that, when the plates were clean, led some to dark corners to sleep with the hushing of the wind, and others to drink mulled wine until our voices had climbed an octave and finally deepened, in the small hours, into whispers. One of the night's final questions, passed around upon faces made golden by candlelight: Was there some way to carry this meal into the rest of our lives?

A week later we were back in our one-bedroom apartment in Vancouver, surrounded by two million other people and staring out the sitting-room window. We have a view of a parking lot and two perpetually overloaded Dumpsters. It was as good a place as any to contemplate the statistic. The number just kept turning up: in the reports that Alisa and I read as journalists; in the inch-long news briefs I've come to rely on as an early-warning system for stories that would, in a few months or a few years, work their way into global headlines. According to the Leopold Center for Sustainable Agriculture at Iowa State University, the food we eat now typically travels between 1,500 and 3,000 miles from farm to plate. The distance had increased by up to 25 percent between 1980 and 2001, when the study was published. It was likely continuing to climb.

I didn't know any more about it than that. It was enough. Like so many other people, Alisa and I had begun to search for ways to live more lightly in an increasingly crowded and raggedy-assed world. There is no shortage of information about this bright blue planet and its merry trip to hell in a hand-basket, and we had learned the necessary habit of shrugging off the latest news bites about "dead zones" in the Gulf of Mexico or creatures going extinct after 70 million years—70 *million years*—on Earth. What we could not ignore was the gut feeling, more common and more important than policy makers or even scientists like to admit, that *things have gone sideways.* That the winter snow is less deep than it was when we were children, the crabs fewer under the rocks by the shore, the birds at dawn too quiet, the forest oddly lonesome. That the weather and seasons have become strangers to us. And that we, the human species, are in one way or another responsible. Not *guilty,* but responsible.

The gut feeling affects people. I received a letter once, as a journalist, from a young man who had chained himself to a rail-ing in a mall on the biggest shopping day of the year in America, the Saturday after Thanksgiving, and set himself on fire to protest rampant consumerism. He survived, barely, and was or-dered into mental health care, but all of his opinions were of a kind commonly held by some of the most lucid and admired ecologists and social theorists of our times. A friend of mine, a re-lationship counselor, told me of a couple whose marriage was being tested by a disagreement over the point at which the world's reserves of cheap petroleum will surpass maximum pro-duction and begin to decline. Concerned for his child's future in an "end of oil" scenario, the husband, an otherwise typical health-care provider, wanted to go bush, learn how to tan buck-

skins, teach their boy to hunt and forage. The wife, equally concerned for the child, preferred everyday life in a society where
carbonated soda is the leading source of calories in the diet of the
average teenager and the *New England Journal of Medicine* reports
that, owing to obesity and physical inactivity, the life spans of
today's children may be shorter than those of their parents. So
who's crazy?

A more typical response is the refusal to purchase an enormous, fuel-inefficient SUV. Alisa and I had made that choice.
Yet, as the Leopold Center numbers seemed to suggest, we had
no cause to feel holier-than-thou. Each time we sat down to eat,
we were consuming products that had traveled the equivalent
distance of a drive from Toronto, Ontario, to Whitehorse, Yukon
Territory, or from New York City to Denver, Colorado. We were
living on an SUV diet.

"I think we should try eating local food for a year."

We were at the breakfast table when these words came out of
my mouth. Alisa did not look up at me as though I were insane.
We had begun to do these kinds of things, insuring the car in
the summer only and getting through the winter by bicycle; or
living part of each year in a northern hideaway where the "emergency procedure" was to wave your arms in front of a passing
freight train and then sit tight and wait—the *following* train was
the one that would stop.

Besides, I do all the cooking.

Alisa had a pensive look on her face. "It might not even be
possible," she said. A long pause settled between us. "What
about sugar?"

She knew immediately, I think, that she had lost the argument. What about sugar? Well, I had learned one or two things about sugar over the previous year, while researching a book set in the Dominican Republic. The journey had taken me through the *bateys,* the shanties inhabited by mainly ethnic Haitian sugar workers, certainly some of the world's poorest people. One afternoon I went out with a nun to pick up an elderly cane-cutter; there was a space for him in the old folks' home that had been set up by the Catholic sisters. We drove past walls of green cane stalks to a clearing with patched-together tin shelters and one-room concrete shacks. The man was leaning against a wall, literally holding himself together with his hands. He had worked so hard and for so long that his hip socket had worn out, and he could not walk without pressing the femur into place. I carried his bag, which contained everything he had to show for a lifetime of labor. It was a schoolchild's backpack, with a broken zipper. Staring out at the men cutting cane as we departed, he said into the air, "Hungry. I've been hungry all these years."

I had taken on the irritating habit, whenever Alisa came to me with some complaint that I considered overly modern and urban, such as the effects of rainfall on suede or a pinched nerve from talking too long on the phone, of saying that I would make sure to let them know all about it in the bateys.

I arched an eyebrow in Alisa's direction. The question of sugar was a reminder of why I wanted to try this local-eating experiment in the first place. It isn't only that our food is traveling great distances to reach us; we, too, have moved a great distance from our food. This most intimate nourishment, this stuff of life—where does it come from? Who produces it? How do they treat their soil, crops, animals? How do their choices—my choices—affect my neighbors and the air, land, and water that surround us? If I knew where my food and drink came from, would I still want to eat it? If even my daily bread has become a mystery, might that total disconnection be somehow linked to the niggling sense that at any moment the apocalyptic frogs might start falling from the sky?

"We'll use honey," I said to Alisa.

"Yeah," she replied doubtfully. "Honey."

What, though, was eating locally? We'd signed up with a company that delivered a weekly box of organic produce to our apartment. For a time we tried to order only "local" foods—products from British Columbia and neighboring Washington State. The delivery company, a very West Coast kind of operation, included on its invoices a tally of our products' average "food miles," or the distance they had traveled to reach our doorstep. Sometimes the average was as low as 250 miles. Sometimes, though, it closed in on 1,000. North Americans live in enormous landscapes. As the writer Wade Davis noted of just one great northern plateau in our part of the world, "you could hide England here and the British would never find it."

We were familiar with the "ecological footprint" model developed by the bioecologist Dr. William Rees of the University of British Columbia. The concept is simple enough: punch in a basic accounting of your housing, along with your transportation, diet, and energy-use habits, and Rees's computer program will approximate the number of acres' worth of the world's resources you consume in a year. That acreage is the size of your ecological footprint. To drive the point home, the software then alerts you to the number of Earths we human beings would need if everyone on the planet consumed in the same way you do. It's usually a shocker—nine planets is a typical figure for a standard-issue North American.

Interestingly, Rees traces the roots of his eco-footprint brain wave to a single meal on his mother's family farm in southern Ontario when he was a boy. It was the early 1950s, "the pre-tractor days," so some thirteen brothers, sisters, parents, cousins, aunts, and uncles were gathered on his grandmother's country porch for a workday lunch on a July afternoon. Young Bill looked down at his food and had a kind of epiphany. The baby carrots, the new potatoes, the fresh lettuce—there wasn't a single foodstuff on that plate that he hadn't had a hand in growing. It was a feeling, he remembers, like a rush of cold water being poured down his back. He was riveted. He was so excited he couldn't eat his lunch.

It was, like, everything was *connected*.

Rees's footprint calculator asks its users to estimate the average distance their food travels, giving as its lowest option "200 miles or less." When Alisa and I looked at a map, however, that distance didn't make sense. A 200-mile line, drawn outward from our apartment in Vancouver, might leap mountain ranges, cleave river valleys, enter landscapes so different from ours that if you took a stranger from one to the other, he might imagine he'd entered another country. Our West Coast landscape is defined by lushness and rain; 200 miles to the northeast the prairie is studded with prickly-pear cactus, and tumbleweeds roll along the shoulder of the highway.

Poring over the map that day, we considered, for the first time ever, the boundaries of the place in which we live. From the east flows the mighty Fraser River, the most productive salmon river in the world and, almost miraculously, never dammed. The great alluvial plain of the river, known simply as the Fraser Valley, widens from the foot of the Coast Range to the vast estuary where the fresh water meets the salt. Every inch of that valley is freighted with a million years' worth of soil perfect for the plough. Just to the north of the delta is the city of Vancouver, sprawling over two inlets and, increasingly, everything else besides. Farther north is Howe Sound, a classic fjord with canyons at its head that reach to the town of Pemberton, famous for its potatoes. There, again, closes a labyrinth of mountains. Look to the south, and it is just 38 miles to the Washington border and the Nooksack and Skagit lowlands, riverine landscapes less grand in scale than the Fraser Valley, but still places where a person has no trouble feeling small. Here, across an international border that wasn't drawn in ink until 1872, the Coast Range is known as the Cascade Mountains, peaks that wall in the farms between the summits and the sea. To the west is the ocean. But not the open ocean, not yet. The coast here is sheltered by Vancouver Island, itself the size of Vermont and hoary with forest. Between the mainland and the huge island are the Strait of Georgia, Juan de Fuca Strait, and Puget Sound, together forming a gulf that some now call the Salish Sea after the name used by the Indian nations who have lived on its shores for millennia. By any name, it is jeweled with islands, some Canadian and some American, but most of them checkered with small farms and orchards. On the southern tip of Vancouver Island is the city of Victoria, capital of British Columbia, surrounded by farm holdings and precocious vineyards. At last, on the island's far western shore, roars the wild, open Pacific.

All of this, blessed with mild winters and rain that falls as if someone once prayed too long and too hard for it to come.

We drew it into a circle and measured the distance. It was, almost to perfection, 100 miles. The 100-Mile Diet. I stood up from the map and caught Alisa's eye. "This might turn out to be too easy," I said.

We chose the first day of spring to begin what we hoped would be a year-long experiment. Like urbanites everywhere, we imagined that, at the stroke of midnight on the last day of winter, fresh green shoots would burst from the earth to nourish us. The fact that a woolen sky and bone chill still pressed down on the city could hardly worry us.

We had a single ironclad rule: that every ingredient in every product we bought had to come from within 100 miles. On the other hand, we are of that generation that mistrusts dogma, doctrine, and ironclad rules in general. We allowed ourselves what we called "the social life amendment." Should friends have us over for dinner, or working life lead to a business lunch at a Thai restaurant, we would not hesitate. We were off the hook, too, when we traveled—even the Koran allows travelers a break from the fast of Ramadan—unless we were able to buy our own groceries and prepare our own meals. When traveling, we were also free to bring home products from within 100 miles of wherever we were. That said, we could not plan a trip to Hawaii because of a pineapple craving.

Puritanism was not the goal, and neither was life as a couple of back-to-the-landing hermits. Our purpose was a lifestyle experiment that challenged us to explore, and explore deeply, the idea of local eating. There was one final point that would ease us into the diet. We allowed ourselves to use up whatever nonlocal products we had in the house on the day that we stepped cold-turkey into 100-mile shopping. And so, when the morning of March 21 dawned sodden and gray, we had our first fight.

There was Alisa, spooning cocoa into a mug. Certain friends had snorted that the 100-mile diet would be easier for Alisa and me because neither of us drinks coffee, which wreaks havoc on our respective nervous systems. We had found a gentler replacement in hot chocolate, though, and a morning caffeine hit by any other name is still a morning caffeine hit.

"We have to start this clean," I said firmly. "A 100-percent-local breakfast."

"It's in the rules," she said.

"But I'm not having any."

"And I am."

"You can't have any if I'm not having any." I could hear the eight-year-old in my voice, but couldn't seem to control him. Every spoonful she took without me was a lost share in the precious cargo. "It wouldn't be fair."

"There's no 'you can't if I'm not' in the rules," she snapped back.

"You're robbing me of future hot chocolate!"

There was some mutual sulking over plates of potato fritters.

For the inaugural dinner, we had invited two good friends: Ron, whose interest in the arcane politics of food had led him to work cooking healthy dinners alongside heroin and crack addicts on the desperate streets of Vancouver's Downtown Eastside; and Keri, who is married to Ron and may be the first genuine green thumb I have ever known. Keri could spit a tomato seed into a dirty ashtray and harvest pendulous, sweet-to-bursting beef-steaks precisely eighty days later. Not even she had any sprouts coming up yet in her garden, though.

We had some shopping to do. The nearest grocery to our house, just three blocks away, is what once was called a "super-market" but is now on the small end of mid-size. The morning was gray enough that the bank of front windows glowed, making even the parking lot seem cheery. I'd never entirely lost that childhood sense of importance that comes with the submissive giving-way of an automatic door, and today we were paying more than the usual attention to such familiar details, the way the shelves stood just as tall as our reach, the corridors of brightly packaged products incessantly refreshed.

All of it, gone. There was nothing there for us. Nothing. All of that plenty, vanished in an instant of cockeyed imagination. It would be a year without ice cream. A year without salad dressing. A year without all-purpose flour, soup mix, olives, olive oil, Miracle Whip. Without ketchup, Cheerios, Peek Freans Fruit Cremes, peanut butter, Rip-L-Chips, Philadelphia cream cheese, Tabasco sauce, Campbell's Chunky New England Clam Chowder, creamed corn, Minute Maid orange juice, no-name cola, Eggos, bulk pine nuts, Orville Redenbacher's popcorn, chipotle peppers, High Liner Multigrain Tilapia Fillets. The shopping aisles represented a kind of miracle. They were the terminus of a quarter-century of progress from a postwar North American diet that defined shrimp cocktail as exotic and offered maybe six brands of beer; they were a paean to a decade of global trade deregulation that finally collapsed as the world's richest nations refused to sincerely reduce the gross subsidies to—what else?—their farms and their farmers. A single supermarket today may carry 45,000 different items; 17,000 new food products are introduced each year in the United States. Yet here we were in the modern horn of plenty, and almost nothing came from the people or the landscape that surrounded us. How had our food system come to this?

We finally turned up our first few food choices in the produce department. Crimini mushrooms and potatoes from the Fraser Valley farmlands, perhaps 50 miles away. There was also a handful of greenhouse red peppers and tomatoes; later we found bottles of local milk. A trip to Capers Community Market, a premium grocery renowned for organic food, was only marginally better. Capers is a small chain store with what passes for venerable roots in a city as young as Vancouver; the flagship store opened its doors twenty years ago, staffed by the kind of people who called themselves "capricots" and felt okay about occasionally being paid in food. Since then, Capers has been subsumed into Wild Oats Markets, Inc., the Boulder, Colorado–based natural-food empire that today reports annual sales of over $1 billion. The produce manager still has dreadlocks and rides a bike to work, however, and blue stickers had recently begun to identify locally grown fruit and vegetables. Of course, this was the first day of spring. There was a sale on Happy Planet Organic Smoothies and Soyco Rice Shreds, but not a lot local on offer.

Ron called in the afternoon. "We're going to be a little bit late," he said.

"That's probably a good thing," I replied.

"Can we bring anything?"

I laughed.

At 7:30 p.m., the table was set in what a real estate agent would call our "dining nook." We had, through a comprehensive search of our district's grocers and specialty shops, come up with quite a spread. For the salad, slices of greenhouse cucumber from the Fraser River delta, some 15 miles away. Each was capped with a slaw of winterkeeper organic carrots from Friesen Farm, legendary for its salad mix and located a comfortable 30 miles from where we were sitting, and beet and kohlrabi from our own community garden plot, precisely a quarter-mile away. Steamed kale, also from our garden. Spring salmon, which the fellow in the fish shop assured us was "local," though in fact it was caught off the west coast of Vancouver Island, near the outer limit of our self-imposed entrapment. I fried the fish in unsalted organic butter from a dairy whose cows we'd seen placidly free-ranging while we were cycling on a Fraser River island (21 miles away), infusing it with sage leaves from a plant on our balcony (zero miles). On the side, fritters of organic, free-range eggs (57 miles) and grated potato (99 miles) and turnip (30 miles), each one slathered in organic yogurt (15 miles) and sprigs of anise, which grows around the neighborhood like a weed. The only nonlocal product on the table was the salt in the shaker, from a bagful we had bought weeks earlier that came from Oregon, a few hundred miles away.

"I have a feeling we're going to be eating a lot of potatoes," said Alisa, as she tucked into her third potato-centric meal of the day.

"Ah, but think of how they'll change with the seasons," said Ron, who I suspect is an actual optimist. Even his last name, Plowright, has a can-do, family-farm lilt, though it's also undeniably pornographic. And indeed, his reddish, muttonchop sideburns bring to mind both blue-movie stars and *The Old Farmer's Almanac.* "Think of how excited you'll be to see the first baby potatoes. They'll be like jewels to you. They'll taste like nothing you've ever eaten before."

Keri, not an optimist, looked at Ron as though he were crazy. She looked at all of us as though we were crazy.

For dessert, triangles of warmed organic brie from Salt Spring Island in the Strait of Georgia (37 miles), topped with frozen blueberries from the exurban town of Agassiz (74 miles), drizzled with a cranberry juice (74) and honey (14) reduction. To drink, a bottle of white wine (32) and four glasses of a 7-percent-alcohol hard apple mead in a style called "cyser," presumably because that is how a very drunk person pronounces the word "cider." It came from the Cowichan Valley, about 59 miles away on Vancouver Island, from the appropriately named Merridale cidery. The average distance from farm to plate for the entire meal? About 43 miles, an improvement of 1,457 on the Leopold Center's more conservative statistics.

"Jesus, you guys," said Ron, as he pushed back from what was inarguably a feast, a cornucopia, a horn-of-freaking-plenty. "That was amazing."

"How will we ever survive?" I mused, cradling my belly.

And we allowed ourselves this moment of happiness. Because the grocery bill for that single meal had come to $128.87. Alisa was polite enough to wait until our company had left to say the obvious. "This might not even be possible."

This is the part where some childhood memory is supposed to lift me above all doubt and equivocation. Like the time when I ran through the wind-rippled fields to my grandfather as he worked the soil with his old tractor. I handed him his brown-bag lunch, and he smiled and pulled me up onto his knee. Together we steered into the shade of an orchard, grandpa carrying me on his shoulders to reach for two perfect, sun-dappled peaches . . .

But no. There isn't any moment. I was raised with three brothers on a healthy but suburban diet, with more shredded wheat and less chocolate milk than I would have liked. We had nearly a quarter-acre of garden that I raided for strawberries but resented weeding. I have my share of fond recollections of family and food, but I also remember how, as a boy, I would inhale my dinner so I could get away from my fighting parents; I remember my mother working too hard to feel *The Joy of Cooking.* The smell of fresh-baked cinnamon buns on the weekends wasn't enough to keep our family together. Food is not, to me, the hearth of kinship or the storehouse of sweet memories. It has never been sacred ground.

Can I admit, then, that a part of me silently questioned my

own idea for a year of eating locally? That the essential pointless-
ness of such a gesture is not lost on me? I am acutely aware that
efforts like the 100-mile diet are readily dismissed as "the new
earnestness," which is currently enjoying a very temporary cool,
and I am not deluded enough to feel that I'm *making a difference*
or *being the change I want to see in the world.* Both of these contem-
porary platitudes contain kernels of truth, but both are also
overwhelmed by stark realities. I have traveled these ethical
pathways in one way or another for twenty years now, choosing
to ride a bicycle in homicidal traffic, to reuse my tinfoil and
plastic bags as though I lived in the Depression, to shop little
and buy less. It doesn't make me feel "good." It makes me feel
like an alien. As I pedal through another midwinter rainfall, virtually every indicator of global ecological health continues to
worsen, from biodiversity to energy consumption, and my *being*
has done little to *change* the world. My actions are abstract and
absurd, and they are neither saving the rain forests nor feeding
the world's hungry.

Most of my acquaintances explain away these compulsions of
mine as guilt, the environmentalist equivalent of the hair shirt.
(Most of my friends, incidentally, are similarly compulsive.) But
I don't consider myself guilty, and I've never been quick to wag
the finger of shame. I have groped around for a better hypothesis, and the closest I've come, oddly enough, brings me back to
northern British Columbia and the place where the 100-mile
diet idea took root.

In 1966 the writer Edward Hoagland left New York City
to wander the wilder frontiers of my province, for reasons he
was unable to explain even to himself. It was an experiment, I

suppose, in much the same way that choosing to eat locally is an experiment. At one point Hoagland settled for a time not at all far—about 40 linear miles—from the shack on the Skeena River where Alisa and I had wondered what to do with a moldering cabbage. He returned to New York with the question that might be the only explanation for how our own grand adventure got started. "The problem everywhere nowadays turns on how we shall decide to live. Neither the government leaders nor the demographers have been able to supply an answer."

And he repeated the question, more plainly:

"How shall we live?"

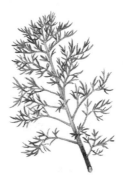

⇥❋ POTATO AMUSE BOUCHE ❋⇤

1 LARGE BEET, PEELED

1 LARGE MASHING POTATO, PARED AND CUBED

3 TBSP BLUE CHEESE

1 TBSP UNSWEETENED APPLESAUCE

1 TBSP BUTTER

SLICE BEETS INTO $\frac{1}{4}$-INCH-THICK ROUNDS. STEAM UNTIL TENDER THROUGHOUT AND SET ASIDE. BOIL POTATO UNTIL SOFT. STRAIN, RESERVING 1 CUP OF COOKING LIQUID. MASH WITH BLUE CHEESE, ADDING COOKING LIQUID AS NEEDED TO ACHIEVE A CREAMY CONSISTENCY. SPOON BALLS OF POTATO MIXTURE ONTO A COOKIE SHEET AND ROAST ON THE HIGHEST RACK IN THE OVEN UNTIL GOLDEN. MEANWHILE, MELT BUTTER IN A SMALL SAUCEPAN. ADD APPLESAUCE AND STIR TOGETHER OVER LOW HEAT. CUT BEET SLICES INTO TRIANGLES OR HEARTS, OR LEAVE AS ROUNDS. PLACE A POTATO BALL IN THE MIDDLE OF EACH BEET SLICE. DRIZZLE WITH APPLE BUTTER. SERVE IN THE CENTER OF A VERY LARGE PLATE, ALONE AND A LITTLE HEARTBREAKING.

APRIL

LONGING IS LIKE THE SEED / THAT WRESTLES IN THE GROUND
EMILY DICKINSON

There are two sides to every story, and here's mine on how this all began: James always carries things one step further than your typical person. If he commits to riding a bicycle, he rides even in the North Pacific monsoons of December that obscure vision, that freeze your bones. If, as he did when he was a twenty-one-year-old rock climber, he decides to impress his new love interest with his strength and bravery, he hangs off the outside edge of a seventeen-story balcony. If he decides that materialism is a problem in modern society, well, he won't shop. It's embarrassing at times. Like when the soles of his favorite brown shoes had worn into stubby flaps. One afternoon, as he dug in his pocket to give a panhandler some change, the guy said, "Keep it, man. You look like you need it."

After that he bought a new pair of shoes.

So when James said, as we sat eating breakfast in our dining nook beneath an often-mocked painting of earnest ducks, "Let's eat only local food for one year," my arm froze before I could deliver my forkful of syrup-slathered French toast to my mouth. His pale blue eyes with their sweet Finnish tilt looked so seriously at me, so expectant, excited, hopeful—and challenging.

Is this going to be one of those hanging-off-balconies, shoes-that-hoboes-pity kind of projects? I asked myself.

That afternoon, though, I found myself flipping through the gardening catalog, pausing on vegetables I'd never considered before. French Breakfast Radish (a radish for breakfast?), an old-fashioned or "heritage" variety that can be planted in March on the West Coast and matures in twenty-five to thirty days. Komatsuna, a Japanese green also known as mustard spinach; sow in March, twenty-one days to maturity. Arugula, thirty to forty days. I could feel myself giving in.

The next thing you know, I was eating a whole lot of latkes. That first, overpriced 100-mile meal was, as they say, "unsustainable," and within days we had homed in on the humbler cold-weather harvest: root crops and hardy winter greens. James is the household cook—so good in the kitchen that I've never had an incentive to try—and bore the burden of creating the new menus. Breakfast might be potato and parsnip fritters made with free-range eggs. For lunch, colcannon, the sexed-up name the Irish give to mashed potatoes with kale or cabbage. He would try to surprise me at dinner: some golden rutabaga, maybe, with grated raw beet and goat cheese salad, and sunchokes scalloped in milk. For those who've never seen or eaten the sunchoke, also known as the Jerusalem artichoke or sunroot, it's a tuber native to North America. It looks like ginger. It tastes, well, like a nutty little potato.

These are the foods that keep well in storage, or the tough ones that continue in the soil, shrugging off the winter. In the first weeks we ate a lot of borscht. It was comfort food, perfect for the season, but with a touch of melancholy. I got the recipe from my former pen pal Mary, a sweet grandmother in her seventies with one or two peculiarities that got her into trouble with the law: she stripped naked in public sometimes, and set things on fire. Her exhibitionism and tendency to arson were acts of protest motivated by her faith. Mary was a radical "Sons of Freedom" Doukhobor, a Christian sect of pacifists who reject state government and construct self-sufficient vegetarian communities. The "Dukes," as they once were called by the hostile popular press, came to Canada from Russia in 1898, funded by the proceeds of Tolstoy's final novel, *Resurrection,* and hoping for a final refuge from persecution. In the 1920s, however, the Canadian government reneged on its promise that the Doukhobors could keep property in common and would never have to serve in a war. Decades of resistance and arson followed. I met Mary when I was a student journalist, and she started writing to me from the prison where she'd been a regular presence for the past fifty years. Jarringly, she sent me her recipe for borscht in the middle of a thirty-day fast behind bars. Her political protest didn't stop her from dreaming of the tastes of home.

I hadn't heard from Mary since she got out of jail ten years ago. I had no idea where she was now—the Sons of Freedom don't list themselves in the phone book. The feelings evoked by every bowl of borscht, then, were paradoxical. The soup softened any feelings of self-pity, but at the same time reminded me that James and I were eating the foods of austerity. Borscht belonged to the long winters of the nineteenth-century Russian steppes, flavored by bone-chilling wind, a steel sky, and oppression. Beets, cabbage, potatoes—these days a winter diet was as anachronistic as the fading Doukhobor culture. "War vegetables," James called them. As we slowly revealed our 100-mile diet experiment to friends and acquaintances, they would often make the same automatic connection. First would come the nod of sage approval, and then, "Ah, you're eating like our grandparents did."

And I would think, "Not *my* grandparents."

For months I had been worrying about my grandmother. I was used to thinking of her on the move; if she could persuade a friend to go to Machu Picchu or the Great Wall of China, she was content. Golfing in California would do as second best. Then, last winter, she fell and broke her neck at the age of eighty-four. While she had graduated to a simple neck brace from a horrible "halo" screwed directly into her skull, she still showed no signs of getting out of bed.

Living in a cramped urban apartment makes it hard to hang on to reminders of everyone who is important to you, and I've found books to be the most efficient system. I crossed the ten feet from the kitchen table to the living room bookshelf and reached up for *The Good Housekeeping Cook Book,* a World War II edition that my grandmother had relied on as a young wife and mother. Here and there she had made notes on its pages, adjusting the amount of salt in a pickle recipe, or rewriting the ingredient measures for a pumpkin pie where the paper had worn through from frequent use. I lingered longingly over that page.

In the days leading up to our 100-mile diet, I had never stopped to consider that flour might not be available. Most of the foods we had to do without were obvious enough—like oranges and mangoes—but others seemed like whims of an invisible economy. Our first shopping trips around town revealed that there were no local cooking oils; we would have to get by with butter. Vancouver's sugar factory got its sugar beets from the Prairies and raw cane from the tropics. No one seemed to grow tea around here or, James realized with despair, barley for beer. I mournfully placed back on the shelf the bags of rice labeled PRODUCT OF THAILAND or PROUDLY GROWN IN CALIFORNIA; we used to eat rice nearly every day. There was no pepper and no salt. No salt? It was only the staple seasoning of the entire world. I could taste it in the air, but couldn't buy it in a box. We would have to ration the two-pound bag of Oregon sea salt that was already in our cupboard. We dubbed it "sinner's salt."

More than anything, I kept coming back to the wheat. It is the staff of life, present at every meal in one way or another. I had assumed it grew everywhere, too. But of course: my mental images of late-afternoon light falling on golden fields of grain were all from my childhood on the Canadian Prairies, or from long holiday drives through the American plains. Now I lived in a mountain landscape drenched with rain. My hopes soared when, scouring a health-food store, I found a brown bag labeled Anita's Organic Grain & Flour Mill, which was located about 60 miles up the Fraser River Valley. I called as soon as I got home, and reached Anita herself. She gently explained that her nearest grain suppliers were 800 miles away by road. She sounded sorry for me. Would it be a year until I tasted a pie?

Meals were the all-important social glue to my grandmother. My family went over to her house every Sunday for about fifteen years, from the time she moved to the city of Victoria to be near my mother, her eldest daughter, until she moved into a senior's apartment with no kitchen four years ago. There were also the grand New Year's, Easter, Thanksgiving, and Christmas feasts for which she and my mother had alternated as lead chef, but always companionably helped each other all day. Before each of these holiday meals we would sing our family grace:

Be present at our table Lord
Be here and everywhere adored
These creatures bless and grant that we
May feast in paradise with Thee. Amen.

My grandmother was religious but my mother was not; this was my only formal communication with God, and it was all about food.

And so, when I was about to move to New York in my early twenties for a five-month magazine internship, I faced cooking for myself for the first time in my life—really, my first try at cooking in any serious way at all. Clearing the table after a Sunday dinner, I asked my grandmother for any suggestions.

"There's my Tuesday-night noodle casserole," Grandma replied. She wrote out the recipe for me in her spidery but elegant script, the kind of handwriting that doesn't seem to exist anymore:

1 8-OZ PACKAGE NOODLES

½ LARGE TIN SALMON

½ PACKAGE ONION SOUP (DRY)

1 TIN CREAM OF CELERY SOUP

SLICED CHEESE (OPTIONAL)

COOK AND DRAIN THE NOODLES. ADD THE OTHER INGREDI-
ENTS. COVER WITH CHEESE SLICES IF DESIRED. BAKE AT 350
DEGREES FOR A HALF HOUR.

—SERVES 4

I couldn't believe what she had written. Given how much care she put into our Sunday meals, I was surprised by how "packaged" this recipe was. Then, in the gravelly voice that always reminded me of 1940s movie stars, my grandmother sprung this one on me: "I never liked to cook."

I guess I take after my grandma. My mother, following the rule that children diverge from their parents, trained to be a dietician and acquired a now-obsolete university degree in "home economics." She disliked the institutional settings she apprenticed in, and never pursued the career, but she always cooked healthy meals for us at home. The nightly dinner plate was anchored by pork chops or chicken, always served with a fresh green salad. Her daily mantra was three-glasses-of-milk, three-glasses-of-milk. Though never a hippie, my mother did pick up some of her generation's back-to-the-land attitude: in the early 1970s we lived on a 132-acre country property where she kept a huge garden, picked rose hips to make jelly, and even kept bees. We moved to the city when I was five, but she still had a backyard garden, and in summer I remember surreptitiously pulling up carrots—the sweetest, most illicit flavor of my youth.

But she never taught my two younger sisters or me how to cook. From the time I was nine, when my father was slowly dying of multiple sclerosis and my mother was his full-time nurse, she had us wash dishes, vacuum, tidy, take out the garbage, clean the bathroom—but never peel potatoes, slice carrots, or knead dough. My father died when I was eleven, and my mother returned to her post of housewife. She never asked us to do a single chore again.

Wherever I go now, I am surrounded by women like me who did not learn the household arts. It may have been a feminist act by our mothers to save us from lives of drudgery. While politics were never explicitly discussed in my family, as a child I developed strong aversions. Learn to type, and you would become a secretary. Learn to cook, and you were doomed to be a housewife. The same spirit likely motivated James's working mother to make her husband and four sons each prepare one dinner a week. Young James quickly left behind his first tentative meals of spaghetti with Ragu sauce and is now a masterful what's-in-the-fridge cook—not a "chef," he'll insist, but a cook. Of course, I'm stuck doing the dishes.

Over the last few years, though, I began to wonder if the more important question wasn't who does the cooking, but what are we eating. It started with apples. All through my childhood, apples always came with a little "B.C." sticker on them, just as, in other places, they might have said "Washington" or "New

York." Red Delicious was king of the supermarket, though I found them pulpy and bland. I don't believe I ever had another kind; I just knew that something didn't taste right. In the 1990s, baby boomers' gourmet ideas reached the grocery stores and, along with bagels and Thai curry paste, new kinds of apples began to appear: Jonagold, Gala, Braeburn, Fuji. I enjoyed this new world of choice, especially when organic apples showed up on the shelves. Organics came to occupy a peak of food morality for me. The word sounded good for the earth and for my health. Then I began to notice these apples were often from New Zealand, which made me marvel. I've been to that distant country once in my life—I remember an uncomfortable twenty-four-hour plane journey—because my aunt lives there. Now my food seemed to be covering that distance a few times a week.

Unlike wheat, though, apple trees are a familiar sight in Vancouver backyards—the city is at the point of a triangle formed by the great apple-growing regions of the Okanagan in British Columbia and the confluence of the Yakima, Wenatchee, and Columbia rivers in Washington. Yet these apples were being edged out of local supermarkets. What happened to the fruits of our region? Don't apples store for months if kept cool?

It was time for a closer look at the ugly statistic about the distances that food now travels from farm to plate. I sat down at my 1950s wooden desk; my "office" is only two feet from my bed, making it the world's shortest commute. I phoned Rich Pirog, the food systems program leader for the Leopold Center at Iowa State University, and the man responsible for the statistic. The explanation for long-distance eating, he said, comes down to two familiar words: cheap oil. It might not seem that way when we're filling up with gas, but even if you ship a tomato from Florida to the Midwest, the transportation costs are only 6.3 percent of the retail price. According to a 2001 study for which Pirog was the lead author, shipping food nationally uses *seventeen times* more fuel than a regional food system.

Pirog has seen his 1,500-mile statistic reach far and wide through the media. But look more closely, he said. The study only covered fresh produce, not packaged goods that each can contain a laundry list of ingredients from across the continent and around the world. What's more, the study only measured the distances the foodstuffs had traveled *within* North America. A more recent Leopold Center examination of a humble container of strawberry yogurt, processed and sold in Iowa from Iowa milk, required endless patience phoning processors and producers, along with a whole new mathematical formula. The "weighted total source distance" turned out to be 2,216 miles— without considering the plastic container, foil, or box. Meanwhile, international imports form a greater and greater part of our daily nourishment. In 1970, Pirog noted, only 21 percent of America's fresh fruit was imported. By 2001 the figure had nearly doubled. Building on the Leopold Center methodology, new research into the "food miles" traveled by produce and a few simple processed foods is likely more accurate. The public health department of Waterloo, Ontario, puts the typical distance from farm to plate at more like 2,500 miles—the distance from San Francisco to Miami by direct flight, or, more interestingly, from London, England, to Baku, Azerbaijan. In other words, worlds apart.

Pirog confirmed that the number is only increasing. "China wants to be the main produce provider for the world," he said. The implications are huge. Cheap Chinese labor will produce mountains of "bargain" lettuce to be shipped by freighter around the world. More and more, North American consumers will eat produce from distant places they will never visit, though they might easily have grown the vegetables in their own backyards. In fact, they might be eating that imported produce at exactly the same time that it's growing just a few miles away. This is called "redundant trade"; consider, for example, the fact that international strawberry imports to California peak during that state's strawberry season.

All that food comes with a hidden price. The economic term for these invisible costs is "externalities," which *The Economist* magazine refers to as a form of "market failure." I had a ready example lodged uncomfortably in my mind. Reading Marc Reisner's *Cadillac Desert: The American West and Its Disappearing Water*, I had learned that California built 1,200 major river dams en route to becoming the world's number-five agricultural producer. Some California rivers are drained nearly dry by the time they reach the coast—85 percent of all water in the state is used for agricultural purposes. In exchange for this staggering ecological assault, I am able to buy California lettuce year-round. I don't have to pay for the dams, the wild places given over to reservoirs and farms, and the resulting decimation of species from chinook salmon to the least Bell's vireo to all the plants of the bunchgrass prairies. Furthermore, I don't chip in on the cost of cleaning water wrecked by the pesticides and herbicides used in intensive industrial farming; the health-care costs of water

pollution; the greenhouse gas emissions produced in the manu-
facture of nitrogen-based fertilizers, which may also have been
shipped from the other side of the world; or the fossil-fuel emissions, five times greater per mile than those from a cargo truck if
the produce came to town by refrigerated jumbo jet, as it increasingly does. The list goes on. By the time you're eating a
salad the backstory is pretty bleak—what economists who cal-
culate externalities now call the "true cost" of a product. Meanwhile, down at the grocery store and outside the world of theory,
the lettuce stays cheap.

But as one week turned into two and three on our 100-mile
diet, I began to wonder how long I would have to go without
tossed salad. Where were the fresh green shoots? Our local farmers' markets wouldn't open until May. I looked despairingly at
the rows of days left on the calendar. Even the local beets were
gone from store shelves now. I wondered if we had done it single-
handedly. Who else eats that much borscht?

As I considered what Pirog had told me, and looked over the
impressive array of studies he had done centering on Iowa, I
realized that the questions he was asking were exactly the same
as those that James and I were suddenly living. No matter that
Iowa was rolling prairie and our landscape was temperate rain
forest, that Pirog was two time zones and 2,000 miles away. The
story of our place was the story of his, and each was a kind
of everywhere. No region feeds itself anymore: we all stand in
reference to the same global food system. Wherever you may
choose to go, the same trucks zip across the landscape filled with
the same chicken nuggets or canned cream corn, and the fertile
fields are turned into housing tracts. The lettuce was grown in

Asia and came to port under a Panamanian flag-of-convenience. All is hidden and anonymous.

We could continue to decipher every far-flung product that appeared on our supermarket shelves. Or we could start fresh. We could immerse ourselves in the here and now, and the simple pleasures of eating would become a form of knowing.

My grandmother had a growing list of things she would not eat—onions, garlic, spices, tomatoes, green peppers. For the last few years she had suffered from a chronic and intensifying nausea that no doctor could diagnose. She was five feet seven and now weighed less than 90 pounds.

Her memory, too, was in rebellion, and this was precisely what she had most desperately feared about getting old. It was a terrible thing to witness. In early March my family had taken her to a Mexicali restaurant for her eighty-fifth birthday. I had gone back to Victoria for the occasion, the city where I had lived from age fourteen to twenty-nine until Vancouver beckoned, and the city where I had met James. Victoria is quiet, leafy, content to be accessible only by ferry or by plane, its sense of separation on Vancouver Island heightened by the distant backdrop of the Olympic Mountains of Washington State.

My mother had pushed the wheelchair out the nursing home door, my grandmother grimacing over the jolts from the uneven sidewalk. I tried to keep up a cheerful patter to distract her from the obvious pain. It was only after we'd settled at a table in the restaurant that I realized how impossible the whole experience had become. My mother read the menu out loud over and over, because by the end of it my grandmother would have forgotten

what she had heard. "What's 'pasta'?" she asked finally, and my
heart sank.

Sometimes, though, she would look at me and know exactly
who I was and that she loved me, and that I loved her. Perhaps
she let go of food because her feelings about it were ambiguous.
Since the revelation that she had never liked to cook, I had
learned that, during her decades as a housewife, she had produced an unvarying weekly schedule of meals. It was a revelation
to me that she could both conform and rebel at the same time.
She was a loving mother of four and the wife of an air force offi-
cer, which meant she had to clean her home to literal white-
glove, dust-the-doortops perfection. She was most at ease as
party hostess to the air force brass and their wives. My grandmother had been a stunning beauty, a brunette with large eyes
and high cheekbones, with a figure hovering between curva-
ceous and slender. I could easily imagine her in a satin cocktail
dress with a martini in hand. Even as she became absentminded,
she kept up her era's habit of making wry puns at the dinner
table. She liked to keep things jolly.

The Good Housekeeping Cook Book, then, was a hidden history.
Studying its 981 pages, I realized that its authors assumed complete ignorance on the part of the reader, though for reasons different from mine. There were instructions on how to mash
potatoes, how to boil broccoli, how to fry an egg. The book illus-
trated the great social shift that took place after World War II,
when the idea of the "housewife" took root alongside adver-
tisements for status-indicating "labor saving" devices for the
kitchen. My grandmother had never pictured her own mother in
the kitchen. Her father was a doctor-administrator, and they had

a household servant; she remembered her mother horseback riding, golfing, and painting. I figured I was at least four generations removed from the knowledge of how to can a tomato. I wondered how many other grandmothers would rather reminisce about their champion university women's hockey team or their time studying fashion design in Chicago than bake yet another pumpkin pie.

And yet here I was, suddenly confronted by the urgent reality of food. "Give us this day our daily bread" is not only a spiritual metaphor, but a physical requirement. Three weeks into our local-eating experiment, James and I had eaten the last slice of bread from the refrigerator freezer. I remembered one of my favorite childhood books, *The Long Winter,* and how I had relished Laura Ingalls Wilder's tale of privation. In that homestead year of 1880, seven months of fierce blizzards blocked the train and all food supplies from reaching the Dakota Territory. Wilder's father stemmed the family's starvation midwinter when, cleverly noticing a false wall concealing a grain cache in a neighbor's house, he brought home a bucket of seed wheat that the girls and their mother painstakingly ground into flour in a coffee mill. I had to admit it. I was hungry. Whether boiled, fried, baked, roasted, or mashed, potatoes just didn't have the caloric oomph of bleached white flour.

"Tell it to the bateys," James said over a hash-brown breakfast. We were not starving; this was neither the Long Winter nor the nineteenth-century Russian steppes. We lived five blocks from a fish shop with local salmon, oysters, clams, and mussels. Capers grocery store, while thus far bereft of local spring produce, did have artisan cheeses and organic eggs, and anything we could find we could fry in Fraser Valley butter. Yet my pants were sagging off my hips. It was like an accidental Atkins diet.

"I think your ass fell off," said James as I stood up to clear the table.

"So did yours," I snapped.

A few hours later he popped his head into my office—the bedroom—and asked what I wanted for lunch. It was his little joke. Lunch, we both knew, would be potatoes with whatever else was in a nearly empty fridge.

"I'd kill for a sandwich," I replied.

James paused for a moment. "Okay," he said, "I'll make you a sandwich."

I sat at my desk, curiosity and suspicion aroused. How would he make a sandwich? We had no bread, only a few tablespoons of remnant flour. I had scoured the list of farmers on the local Certified Organic website, which named a single farm that grew wheat. "I tried that last year, but there was no market for it," the farmer had told me over the phone. Another farmer supposedly grew oats. "For animal fodder," he explained. I didn't tell him that soon I'd be ready to fight a goat for its feed.

I was drawn from my thoughts by the sounds of pans clattering and James humming, the oven door slamming. I crept out toward him, but he heard me and roared, "Stay out of the kitchen!" Finally he called me to the table. It was neatly set, as it often is when James feels he has managed something special. He flourished a hand toward what appeared to be a sandwich festooned with a red-tipped deli toothpick. It actually looked beautiful, like something you might see in an upscale restaurant.

Layers of bright red greenhouse peppers and fried mushrooms peeked out beneath delectably oozing goat cheese.

"But what is *that?*" I asked, pointing at the twin slabs, grilled to a golden brown, that bookended the sandwich filling.

"That is the 'bread,' " said James.

A by-now familiar odor was offering hints. "And what is the 'bread' made of, exactly?"

He grinned triumphantly. "Turnips," he said.

I laughed, I nearly cried. It was delicious and I finished it all. But I was still hungry. What kind of year was this going to be, anyway?

I am sorry to do this. I have introduced a character, and I am taking her away. This does not follow the rules of storytelling, but then life rarely does.

It was April 22, a chilly day, clear enough to see into the eastern Fraser Valley where the clouds argue with the sky. "Grandma passed away last night," my mother said, her voice on the phone quieter even than its usual reedy sigh.

Death is always a shock, even when it's someone old—even when that person was in pain, always nauseated, hooked up to an oxygen tank to help her weak lungs breathe. Even when she wanted to go.

Good-bye, dear grandmother.

It was a small funeral in a Victoria chapel. At my grandmother's request, her many friends were absent. Drawn from the corners of the Earth's bioregions and time zones by the lodestone of death: my sister from the grain belt of Saskatchewan, my uncle and aunt and cousins from the boreal forest of northern Alberta, my aunt and uncle from antipodal New Zealand. My mother and stepfather from the home ground, Victoria, and James and me, from across the Strait of Georgia. That was all. No headstone, just the simple burning called cremation. The end of the body. At least she believed in the beyond. She believed that her beloved husband was waiting for her, the man who had drowned in the New Zealand surf in front of her helpless gaze twenty years before; and her dear son Bob, who had suffered from mental illness and committed suicide twenty-five years ago. These two, yes, they were waiting for her. At least, for her sake, I wished it were so. Her final statement was a song: "Somewhere Over the Rainbow."

When we returned to my mother's house, my stepfather, Bryan, a tall, quiet Irishman who was a self-employed gardener, went alone into the yard to plant a young Shannon apple tree. It was a heritage variety, a little like a Granny Smith, he said, originating in once apple-lush Arkansas and brought to a peak of fame in 1904 by winning a World's Fair medal. Bryan invited each of us to shovel a little of the dirt back over the roots, echoes of ashes to ashes and dust to dust, but a more hopeful act. There would be blossoms, and there would be fruit, real apples with flavor and crispness and the timelessness of generations. There would be life from the life-giving earth.

There would be better times ahead. *The Good Housekeeping Cook Book* with its war-vegetable recipes and simple instructions for life on rationed sugar would carry us through. Never mind the borscht, never mind the rain, I would put on a perfect pair of shoes, Paris 1990, and a pink suede peyote-embroidered jacket, Winnipeg 1975, and I would defy James and this diet and I would buy a bar of Denman Island dark chocolate, the best I have ever known, and eat it all.

She never liked to cook.

⇢✵ SPRING SALAD ✵⇠

SPRING GREENS

EDIBLE FLOWERS

½ LB ASPARAGUS

BUTTER

A SPRING SALAD IS NOT A PROCESS, BUT A PATTERN. THE CHOICE OF GREENS DEPENDS DAY BY DAY ON SEASONAL WEATHER. CHOICE IS LIMITED; USE EVERYTHING THAT IS AVAILABLE. CHICKWEED, PIGWEED, BABY SPINACH, ARUGULA, WINTER KALE, ANISE, DILL, DANDELION GREENS, THYME, OREGANO, MIZUNA, TAH TSAI, CORN SALAD, RADISH GREENS, THIMBLEBERRY SHOOTS, WILD ONIONS, STINGING NETTLE LEAVES (STEAMED). TRIM ANY THICK ENDS OFF THE ASPARAGUS. BRUSH SPEARS WITH BUTTER AND ROAST 3 MINUTES AT 500°F. LAY ROASTED ASPARAGUS OVER MIXED GREENS. GARNISH WITH EDIBLE FLOWERS: CLOVER, BORAGE, KALE, VIOLETS, APPLE BLOSSOMS, DANDELION, ANISE, ENGLISH DAISIES, FENNEL, SORREL, MARIGOLDS, ROSE PETALS, LAVENDER, MINT, ROSEMARY, PEA BLOSSOMS. A BLANKET OF FLOWERS.

MAY

Alisa wanted to visit the garden plot, though normally she's quite rational. Or maybe the urge was a kind of excessive rationality. She had opened our seed catalog to the planting chart for the West Coast and showed me everything the book said we could sow. Beets, broccoli, carrots, cilantro, fennel, kohlrabi, leeks, lettuce, onions, parsley, peas, spinach, turnips. See?

I was looking out the window. If spring was in the air, it was the subtlest of seasons. Was the night air slightly less damp and unpleasant than before? Did the windblown rain lie-in at a gentler angle from the sea? It was May Day, for god's sake, and the North Pacific monsoons were unrelenting. It could just as easily have been the first day of December or that most unwelcome of months, February. Alisa had planted by the book beginning even in March, some compulsion driving her out between downpours to seed the mud with arugula, radishes, Japanese greens. Then came the late frost.

"I went by the other day," she said. "There are a few survivors."

We were just out of bed and she was craving a salad; again, a kind of obsession. On one of her sojourns to Vancouver Island in the wake of her grandmother's death, she had come home like a conquering hero with a bag of spring mesclun. The mixed lettuces she held with such an air of triumph had cost $17.99 a pound.

The hunger for fresh vegetables had manifested itself as Alisa watched—*ached* might be the better word—for local asparagus to appear. We had never given thought to "asparagus season," but now paid rapt attention as food writers sang their paeans to the spring vegetable, recalling for the umpteenth time that the eighteenth-century poet Charles Lamb believed the vegetable "inspires gentle thoughts," while Aristotle said it causes erections. The writing, like Alisa's eagerness to get back to the garden, was a reflex reaction. It was May; therefore it was the season of asparagus, of steaming spears whose green is somehow precisely the color of spring, or grilling purple or white varieties to snap-top perfection. Suddenly, asparagus was conspicuously available in the produce departments—where it had been available all winter, just like strawberries and tomatoes and every other unlikely product. The clockwork promotion of the year's traditional first delicacy, the vegetable whose very name is rooted in the Persian word for "sprouts" or "shoots," was a parody of seasonality. It *was* asparagus season, somewhere. In California, according to the labeled bunches in the grocery stores, and in Peru, which is now the world's greatest asparagus exporter. It was not asparagus season along the North Pacific coast. The local product was a no-show due to rain; we heard rumors of mobs jostling for the bunches being sold on the grounds of the famous Asparagus Farm on Vancouver Island, but we couldn't justify a weekend getaway, not even in the name of gentle thoughts and erections.

It was early afternoon by the time we made our way the six blocks to our garden plot. We'd applied for space in a community garden in 2001, after moving into our fifth consecutive apartment without a yard. I never fail, in conversation, to boast of our plot as *the land,* my private joke about a section that measures just three feet by ten. It's not the most "community" of thoughts, but the heaped, bare earth of the narrow gardens, lined up along an abandoned railroad track, always brings to mind televised images of mass graves. I did not say this to Alisa, of course. And in fact there is something cheering about the place, with its madcap fences and trellises. Commercial farmers may hold out for the security of warmer weather, but a community garden is an earthen canvas for mavericks. We rarely see any other gardeners, but even in the snow there will always be a defiant stalk of Brussels sprouts or purple kale.

At first glance, our plot was a confirmation of my mood: a sad little nod to the fact that we'd be eating potatoes-any-style for weeks to come. Looking more closely, though, I could begin to interpret a different message. Radish, komatsuna, even spinach was making a show of frail leaves, each the size of a baby's thumbprint. The garlic shoots were actually robust. The bulbs wouldn't be harvested until autumn, but for the moment the sprouts were a psychological gift. We had planted the individual cloves, what Spanish speakers delightfully call *dientes,* or teeth, in October, then feared for their survival when a rare snowfall struck in December. When the white blanket repealed, we'd found thick, green blades completely unperturbed. Garlic will survive World War IV.

The garden seemed to have the sense that I lacked. Life was stirring here. The seeds, enclosed in muck, had divined some slight warming, a lengthening of days. I let my eyes wander. Sure enough, the ornamental cherry and plum trees were in bloom—magnificent, really, the petals falling against the sea-sky or blowing in damp whirligigs along the curbs.

"There's chickweed," I said. The first small mats of the stuff were forming, the round leaves and thin stalks as delicate as watercress.

"And dandelion," said Alisa. We were stooped now, each of us beginning to pinch up the baby greens. Alisa gathered the dandelion fronds, still more sweet than bitter, and I moved from chickweed to sprays of anise, and from there to sage and borage, and the first peppery leaves of nasturtium. It amounted in all to a handful apiece, but it was a salad, it was the world beginning to brighten to green.

Whatever else they may be, weeds are optimists.

One week later, the first farmers' market began and we faced a revolution. We crossed the city from west to east on the bicycle routes, hopeful but braced for disappointment. Like many people, we had been to farmers' markets occasionally in the past. Too often they seemed first and foremost to offer shiatsu massage, mantelpiece knickknacks, espresso blends, folk music, face-painting. It's fun, in a crazy-hat-day kind of way, but this year we needed the purer ideal: real, farm-fresh food.

We got our wish. At the market entrance, we stopped and gaped. Any circus atmosphere was subsumed in the first harvest, great and green, heaped beneath sun shelters and spilling from the backs of beater vans. The most tender leaves of red lettuce, mustard greens, Swiss chard, tah tsai; emerald frizz of fava bean tips and Bordeaux purple kale. There were no paper-skinned onions or garlic, but we learned in a moment that even those flavors, the foundation of so many meals, have their seasons. For spring there were leeks as fat as ax handles, and garlic tops, called "scapes," each with its single puzzling loop-de-loop crowned with a nascent seed head. Rhubarb—the universal cold-weather "fruit"—and last autumn's frozen blueberries. Free-range organic eggs. "Step on up," said the man known as Big Don, stooped beneath his sunshade. "Everyone is so shy on the first market day." He made his pickles, he explained, not with brine but by fermentation, and they were unlike any pickle I've tasted, with the sharpness of dry wine. We grazed our way from stall to stall, and that alone could have passed for lunch. Almost everything came from the Fraser Valley, the wild nettle tops from Agassiz, the dried chilies—which would replace black pepper in my grinder—from suburban Surrey, not 20 miles away. The only item we bought that day that had even crossed the Salish Sea was a pound and a half of cheese curds.

It was strange. April had been a long month. Now, in an instant, our alien sense of survivalism and self-reliance had vanished; we had reentered a world where goods were on offer. I almost resented the cheery displays of competence and foresight, the shock of what these people had teased from land that could still make your hands ache with cold. Back at the apartment, there was no question: lunch would be some kind of salad. I laid out the new provisions across our two squares of counter space.

For me, cooking always begins with this—the realization that, for the millionth time, there is nothing to do but to start from scratch. I can't recall when I first learned to cook; our family had no television, so my brothers and I grew up with our hands in anything that might be the least bit interesting. My favorite childhood photo shows me, a tiny blond gnome seated on a kitchen counter, with a chef's knife and a malicious grin. I was cooking one dinner a week by the time I was ten years old, and because I was a child, my meal plan never began until the instant that I absolutely had to begin. What was in the refrigerator? What was in the cupboards? A frozen chunk of cod, a can of mushroom soup, garden spinach, some leftover rice. Not bad. Like a musician without classical training, I grew up with no knowledge of the correct way to chop an onion or make *beurre blanc,* and I left the recipe books on the shelf.

Experimentation became my paramount value in the kitchen. When I met Alisa, any remaining restraint disappeared. If every romance can be traced to a spark, ours had to do with food. We had become colleagues, then friends, and finally were sharing a spicy pizza together in a diner run by a Québécoise. She leaned across the counter to look each of us in the eye. "You know what it means when you eat the hot banana peppers?" she said. "It means you are in love." After that, everything seemed preordained. Alisa was impressed that I could cook; I outdid myself trying to impress her. Every dish contained edible flowers, Chinatown oddities, unpronounceable grains. The exuberance finally burst with a catastrophic meal of peaches and green peas in a white sauce rolled in tortillas. To this day, Alisa can't stand the fact that I prefer to honor dinner guests with something untried rather than any predictable standby.

Still, the kitchen remains one of the few areas in my life where I feel competent. Not brilliant, but adequate. I am still that boy: it's dinnertime, let's see what's in the cupboards. It is a moment of free expression. What possible combination of ingredients will work together? What should the meal look like on the plate? Then begins the fluidity of familiar patterns. Garlic skins crack under my fingers, asparagus ends vanish into the stockpot, pine nuts turn to paste under the pestle. It is work, sometimes the only genuinely physical effort in the day.

So I had this 100-mile salad to construct. Our farmers' market haul was loaded with unfamiliar flavors: the sinus heat of peppercress; buttery oyster mushrooms; brown hunks of horseradish root (what the hell would I do with that?). Getting started was easy enough—every kind of green went into a bowl. I had no dressing I could think of, so I would need to add foods with some juices. I work with only three kinds of knife—chef's, paring, and bread—and the big blade made quick, thick slices of the mushrooms. Into hot butter they went, and then I chopped in the garlic scapes. When the mixture began to turn golden, I poured it off onto a plate and cracked two eggs into the fry pan. A plain omelette was cooked and sliced in a minute. I tossed the egg strips into the salad and topped it all with the mushrooms, garlic, and still-warm butter.

Then I paused. We were two months into the 100-mile diet,

but to be honest, our food was still a mystery. None of it had traveled far—potatoes from the Fraser Valley, apple cider from Vancouver Island—but neither had we come much closer to it. We were still relying on food from the grocery shelves, where every product's history is erased. The anonymity is in part a comfort: plastic-wrapped ground beef does little to remind you of the carcass of a cow. At the same time, packaged and processed foods share few of their secrets. From mad cow disease to *E. coli* bacteria to genetically modified ingredients, many North Americans have begun to fear their daily nourishment; 300,000 Americans are hospitalized each year by the food they eat, while fully one-third of Canadians will suffer some kind of food-related illness this year. Even certified organic food is no longer wholly trusted; an $11 billion industry, "organic" foods today may include factory-farmed meat and dairy products, and even synthetic additives or artificial flavors. Organic vegetables are frequently the end products of intensive production methods, and end up on your plate after, say, crossing the continent by diesel truck and passing through a plant that washes 26 million servings of lettuce each week.

My fresh market salad was different. It was human scale. I could relate each item not only to its place but to its specific farm and to the faces of those farmers. Greens from the Langley Organic Growers; eggs from the Forstbauer family farm; garlic scapes from a shy man named Albert. The foods that overflowed our big glass bowl were not only the flavors of spring, but of this particular spring, this unique year with its hard rain and rare glory of sun.

I had long believed that farmers' markets had been a part of the social fabric since time immemorial, but like all market systems, today's North American farmers' markets are an invention. In the mid-1970s there were fewer than 300 officially sanctioned farmers' markets across the United States. The catalyst for change was the Farmer-to-Consumer Direct Marketing Act of 1976, which funded state departments of agriculture to legalize an act that many must have been surprised had been prohibited: the sale of food by farmers to their fellow citizens. California was the first to draft ground rules, in 1978, and America's first dozen modern farmers' markets were launched the following year. Now there are more than 3,100 registered markets and likely thousands more informal ones.

The history of markets is wide-ranging, of course. Mexico's open-air markets really are as ancient as its cultures. Britain, despite a profound cultural bond to its "green and pleasant land," only opened its first market, in Bath, in 1997. Deborah Madison, the local-eating pioneer who founded Greens restaurant in San Francisco, has said that a farmers' market makes a small town out of a big one. It also opens a timeless space in the relentless here and now. The East Vancouver market, which had just revolutionized my attitude about a year of local eating, had seemed so permanent to me. I might have guessed that its history was linked to its backdrop, Trout Lake. I doubt that the small lake holds any trout, but it must have when a man named John Hall walked down a Coast Salish Indian trail in 1863 to "claim" the place. Within a decade a flume from the lake was powering the Hastings Sawmill, the first industry in Vancouver. The mill represented a willful separation from the natural world, and the farmers' market, only now a decade old, is a radical reversal. A farmers' market is an act of re-connection.

My friend Ruben had not been home on market day, but this fact did not stop him from berating us for not bringing him along. Ruben is a part of that subgeneration raised by back-to-the-land hippies, not so much hillbillies as hillwilliams, and his heritage has shaped him, giving him the rare combined abilities both to envisage an object in three dimensions and to build it with consummate skill. Rural life also left him with a love for anything that knocks a few dollars off the standard price, which is why he was folded like a grasshopper into the backseat of our tiny car as we headed out through suburban Vancouver. We were searching for the year's first strawberries.

Like most of us, Ruben is a study in contradictions. Fiercely opposed to consumerism, he is the only person I've known who owns a barber's chair, a parking meter, and a chaise longue. We met as proverbial starving students, and in many ways couldn't have been more different. I am a small man, and the things around me then were also small—a few books, pots and pans, and a whitewater kayak that doubled as furniture. Ruben is a tower of knees and cheekbones, and it could take three days to move his collection of aspirational junk. He was the first person to begin to convince me that *stuff*—tools, buildings, gewgaws, machinery—could have its own poetry and beauty. Now an in-dustrial designer, he is convinced that his craft is dedicated to the production of crap that nobody needs. As if to cement this idea in the core of his values, his working life recently took him to the deregulated trade zones of China, where he witnessed the toxic, soul-deadening, and horribly ironic mass production of feng shui tranquillity fountains. "Systems design," he would tell me, stroking his Salvador Dalí mustache. "What we need now is systems design. Total re-creation of the way we do the things we do."

Such as eating. Ruben had loaned Alisa and me a spare cube freezer from his treasure piles, and it was time to start filling it.

We drove south through the 'burbs, the industrial parks, the outer ring of big-box mosques, Buddhist mega-temples, and ticky-tacky churches. Beyond the tunnel that plunges under the main arm of the Fraser River there was finally the sharp stink of manure and fish meal. We turned onto River Road—there was a time when road names could be that simple—beside the dikes that have tried, not always with success, to hold back the spring freshet for nearly 150 years. We anticipated a 30-mile round trip; according to Ruben, we would burn about one gallon of gas, which, through the magic of combustion, would generate some nineteen pounds of carbon dioxide as exhaust.

It was one of those days. Chocolate-colored cats sunned themselves on the dikes; there were the sounds of blackbirds cronking and new cones snapping open in the warming air. Drivers out here still used their turn signals. "Why have I never been here before?" asked Ruben aloud. The entrance to Westham Island is a single-lane, wood-surfaced drawbridge, the gateway of a place that aspires to sideline itself. The island breathes eccentricity, from the cluster of houseboats that bob in dark river water to the greeting sign that reads

WARNING: THIS ISLAND IS PROTECTED BY
WESTHAM ISLAND GUN CLUB

Alisa and I had "discovered" Westham Island one November several years ago, when we got wind that up to 70,000 lesser snow geese set down on the Fraser and Skagit deltas each winter. It seemed like something we should have noticed. The river mouths, one on either side of the international border, are the endpoints of a 2,500-mile southward journey from Wrangel Island in the Russian arctic. Some of the birds fly the last leg from Alaska in a nonstop, thirty-six-hour, 950-mile push. A concentration of geese shows up on Westham Island because, along with an apparently proactive gun club, the island is home to the Reifel Migratory Bird Sanctuary. And yes, Reifel is pronounced "rifle."

It can be surprisingly difficult to find tens of thousands of pure white birds; we had had our life's first literal wild-goose chase. We'd explored backroads and crept to the edges of sloughs and, finally, by entering a Do Not Enter area of apparent importance to the Department of National Defense, found our quarry. The sight was underwhelming, the geese scattered through a field, both their humorous honking and the scent of their feces carried by the wind. Then the flock lifted from the ground into flight, and it was the cresting of an immense crystal wave beneath the sun.

It is easy to forget just how instantaneously hot a spring day can be. Shirtsleeve weather. There was only one other person, however, in the strawberry fields of the Ellis Farms U-Pick as we turned into the parking area. The recent rains had filled every ditch and swale, and everywhere birds made jungle noises. I think we all felt like children as we scuffed over to the farmer's stand. Behind her back a fact sheet explained that strawberries are related to roses, and that according to lore, a double berry split between two people will make them fall in love. The price list ranged up to 110 pounds. "My god," I breathed, "who would want to pick 110 pounds of strawberries?"

"I would," said Ruben.

"That would be like eating your body weight in berries," Alisa rejoined.

"Exactly my plan!" he said.

The childlike quality of the day accelerated when the woman offered us a little red wagon for our berry pails and sent us out to a stake that had been driven into a row of plants. We were to start picking at the stake, moving up and down the rows, boustrophedon style, and when we were done, to replant the stake so the next gleaner would know what areas had been picked over. It was a pleasing system.

We fell to the task with a natural ease, though it must have been years since any one of us had stood in a farmer's field with mud beneath our feet. Berry picking is a decadent act, and we were not above sampling as we went, knowing as adults that this was a forgivable sin, yet unable to shake the sense of our own naughtiness. Our picking path took us, eventually, past the one other figure among the rows, a man in late middle age who worked with a businesslike briskness.

"A beautiful day," he called out.

"Beautiful," we agreed.

"A little early yet for the berries," he said then. "They're still a bit tart. Better for pie than for eating."

I almost laughed out loud. We were all, I think, taken aback. The man was right, of course—these first berries had yet to be superlatively sun-sweetened to the brink of sweet booziness.

And yet this day! The pleasure of a year's first fruit against your teeth!

"I have found the perfect berry," Ruben announced. He was standing as straight as a scarecrow. Between thumb and index finger he held a berry the size of a plumb bob that deepened its red from cap to tip. He bit into it dramatically. "Oh ho *ho!*" he said in exaggerated pleasure. He handed me the second half.

"Not bad," I allowed, though of course it was outrageously good.

And so passed the time, frog-marching down the rows, filling buckets, loading the wagon, and pausing every few minutes: "I have found the perfect berry." Someone would make the pronouncement, and the others would hoot their derision. "Not firm enough," I might snort. "Too pale," Alisa would declaim. "Too boozy," Ruben might insist. When it came time to weigh the fruit, we had picked 29 pounds.

There is a term for the experience of tugging your little red wagon through a strawberry field, and that term is *traceability*. It's a measure of how close or how distant one is from one's food. The majority of the world's farmers, saving their own seeds and cultivating, raising, and harvesting the plants and animals they themselves eat, have total traceability. They know exactly where their food comes from, and under what circumstances it was produced. On the other hand, there's a person eating an all-dressed hot dog on a Manhattan street corner.

It's no secret that we, as a society, have been losing the traceability not only of our food, but of every aspect of our lives. On any given day, chances are high I will have no idea what phase the moon is in. I cannot reliably list my brothers' birthdates, and I regularly use products that work according to principles that I cannot explain. I suspect I will go through life without meeting any of the people who make my shoes, or even seeing the factories where those shoemakers work. Like many people, Alisa and I have lost all trace of our traceability to community. We've lived five years in the same crappy apartment block, where the rent rises yearly while wages continue to flatline. We've never met the owner of the building, and we know none of our neighbors by name. If we had children, we'd be too busy to get to know their teachers.

Fifty years ago, there was still widespread connection to food and the places that it comes from. In the United States, 40 million people lived in the countryside. Many people kept kitchen gardens, raised chickens, or knew a beekeeper. People fished and hunted, and could differentiate between asparagus season and the squash harvest. Ah, it was a New World idyll, and everyone's hair was neatly combed and the children were all polite.

It is worthwhile to resist the tendency toward moral panic over our dislocation. Consider, for example, that stock eulogy for the wholesome farming life: the claim that legions of modern children have never seen a cow. In a typical example, Illinois congresswoman Ruth Hanna McCormick noisily donated one of her "purebred" cattle to the Chicago Zoo, saying, "It's for the kids who have never seen one. Thousands . . . have seen a rhinoceros and a giraffe, but have never seen a cow." That was in 1929. In perhaps a more accurate survey, a recent chat group on the Flickr website asked, "Who's never seen a cow in real life?" The mostly young, urban, and technologically astute members alternately rolled their eyes or expressed horror at the question. "That is such a weird concept," wrote Becca G. "Are there really people out there who have never seen a cow?" Just one admitted that although he had seen cows, he had never seen "the black and white spotted dairy cows."

Yet there is a reality behind the anxiety. In his economic study *American Agriculture in the 20th Century: How It Flourished and What It Cost,* University of Maryland professor Bruce L. Gardner notes that the United States has lost two-thirds of its farms since 1920. Some of the losses were painfully specific; for example, while nearly a million African-Americans operated farms before the Depression, just 19,000 do so today. The nature of farming changed just as radically. Industrialization, most intensive from 1950 onward, accounted for one-half of America's lost farms. Commercial fertilizer use has more than doubled since World War II, to around 50 million tons per year. There is no way to fathom that kind of figure without mentally stacking blue whales or Sherman tanks. A simpler set of numbers: in 1952, just 11 percent of American corn was treated with pesticides and herbicides; today the statistic is over 95 percent. And on it goes, a pattern of technological apotheosis that marked another milestone with the first genetically modified farm product for human consumption, a cheese enzyme in 1990.

Where once North America's farms were home to the traditional barnyard animals, few are today. The change is quantifiable: for example, just 4 percent of American farms today keep chickens. "The early mornings are strangely silent where once they were filled with the beauty of bird song," wrote Rachel

Carson in *Silent Spring*. On the modern farm, the strange silence is dawn without the rooster's crow.

What made us drift away? In 1920 the rural and urban populations of both the United States and Canada were evenly split. Movement toward the cities stalled with the Depression, but rapidly accelerated with the boom after World War II. The rural customs—self-sufficiency, buying from people you know, shopping catalogs for a few trusted products—could not hold. In the cities, hundreds of brands competed with powerful advertising, while emerging chain stores deployed tactics like selling at a loss to break shoppers' old loyalties. There was no going back to the farm. Agriculture today generates seven times the farm output of a century ago—but with one-third the labor force.

Just 2 percent of Americans now live on farms, and the trend continues globally; last year a UN commission reported that half the world's 6.5 billion people will live in cities in 2007. Most of them, I suspect, will still have seen a cow. Fewer and fewer, however, will have touched one, cared for one, watched one give birth, or seen a cow give milk or its life for our consumption.

We were preparing to leave Westham Island when we saw a sign offering honey and lamb. I turned down the road, then into a carport marked with a second message, HONK FOR SERVICE. Out walked Gail Cameron, slim, bespectacled, wiping a nap from her eyes. Sure, she said, she had honey for sale. She recommended the pumpkin variety.

Pumpkin honey?

Gail pulled a jar from beneath her farmstand and spun a

golden spool onto a dipstick. "Try that," she said. There was the familiar, forward sweetness, but a smokiness seemed to arise from its depths. Then came the taste of pumpkin—not pumpkin itself, but its sugared infusion, like in pie or ice cream. It was unlike any honey I'd ever tasted.

"Do you ever do buckwheat honey?" asked Ruben.

Gail nodded. "Years ago there was a field of it near here."

"My father loved it," Ruben continued. "He grew up in the South and would have it brought up from there. I thought it tasted like cough syrup."

She laughed. "People love it or hate it," she said. "I could never get used to the smell. It smelled like socks."

I had the sensation that a window had opened, expanding the world. I had long been aware that there were different kinds of honey: alfalfa, clover, wildflower. They had always tasted more or less alike to me, none distinctive enough to be a "favorite." More mind-boggling was the idea of a honey so extraordinary in flavor that I actually *might not like it.* The epiphany felt urgent, a gentler version of that first adolescent kiss that tells you there's something good you've been missing out on all your life. I wanted to know these honeys. I wanted to live in this world where I had opinions on the harvests of bees.

"If you're looking for something stronger . . ." said Gail. She dipped into a jar that was a diuretic amber. "Dandelion," she said. "The first honey of the year."

It is not an overstatement to say the flavor exploded in my mouth. Honey is flower nectar that has been concentrated by bees, which beat their wings to evaporate the water and, less appetizingly, regurgitate it as many as 200 times until it is

80 percent sugar. The sweetness of the dandelion honey was immediate, and so was its pungent earthiness, like the smell of good compost. The honey tasted *radically* different. There were floral perfumes and hints of roasted chestnuts and of the bitter white dandelion milk that everyone seems to have sampled as a child. This honey demanded that its taster take a position for or against. It tasted like politics.

"Eech," said Alisa, who considers herself shy. "It's awful."

"What does it taste like to you?" I asked, ready to argue that its muskiness might be an acquired taste.

"Aluminum foil," she replied.

We settled on a jar of pumpkin and another of blueberry, which had a water-light suggestion of ripe berries, and Don and Gail Cameron became our honey suppliers. Don does the actual beekeeping, a hobby he began after retiring from a career on the money-market desk at the Bank of Canada. "I guess I believe that making an abrupt turn in terms of a career or what comes after a career is usually healthy," he says.

There is still an air of casual Friday about him, with his moccasin shoes, tattersall shirt, and silvery hair. Don can talk about honey as a business, but the apiary life has taken him into less pragmatic terrain as well. "There's kind of a foot in the past," he told me. "Beekeeping hasn't changed much for a hundred years, and the essence of it hasn't changed for an *awfully* long time. There's a simplicity to it, and a connection." On the spring day I chatted with him, he led me to bees gathering pollen from a pink clematis, and he knew that it was 17 degrees Celsius, or 63 degrees Fahrenheit, and that the nectar was therefore running, despite the in-flow breeze. As he walks the Westham Island dikes, he's aware in a way that few of us are; he pays attention to what's in bloom, which flowers draw only butterflies, how strong the wind can blow before the burly bumblebees ground their flights. He tastes the seasons in his honeys, what beekeeping author Holley Bishop has called "a sweet, condensed garden in your mouth." It was his bees, Don said, that led him to pumpkin honey. One summer they started hauling in an ochreous nectar, their bodies orange with pollen as if dipped in powdered cheese. The bees had discovered a pumpkin patch. "There's enough to keep you interested—forever," said Don, sounding surprised as the last word popped out of his mouth.

The Camerons' honey had answered a question for us. It was eleven dollars a pound, while sugar was $2.59. Well, we would eat fewer sweets and enjoy them more. Thousands of generations of people had done the same. Sugar plunged below the price of honey only in the mid-1800s. Today a typical North American consumes more than a cup of sugar a day and perhaps two cups of honey a year. Alisa and I would reverse the trend. We would do so knowing our "bee pastures" and the hands of the keeper who, on a hot summer day, can rob his bees so gently that not a single one is killed, so gently that he doesn't even bother to smoke out the hives.

Back in the car, Ruben was thoughtful. "If grocery shopping were always like this, it wouldn't be a chore," he said.

On the other hand, Ruben did not join Alisa and me on our mission to pick up a tubful of wheat. I had placed a call to a farmer named Jim and explained the 100-mile project.

"Well," said Jim, "I'm not growing any wheat this year."

"But you grew some last year?"

"I grew a variety called Red Fife last year as an experimental trial. We tried it out with a few bakers, but there was a problem with too much gluten."

This seemed to me to be splitting hairs. "But you grew wheat?"

"Sure."

"Do you have any left?"

"Tell you what," he said. "There's a one-ton bag of it in my barn. Why don't you just come on out and help yourself to as much as you like?"

"Are you serious?"

We arrived two days later, following his instructions into the Fraser delta and the fields lorded over by the great bald head of Mount Baker, the northernmost of the postcard volcanoes that pop up from Washington to California. The quiet road was lined with trees in old catkins and new leaves. Just as Jim had promised, there was a big old red barn, wind-polished on the corner that tilted into the winter sou'easters. We felt like trespassers. We expected rural dogs, the kind that had chased my wheels on so many childhood bike rides.

The barn was crosshatched with dusty light. "How will we know what we're looking for?" asked Alisa. "What does a one-ton bag of wheat look like?"

I didn't need to answer. I had turned to face a plumped-out sack nearly as tall as I am and spotlighted by a pale but heavenly ray. Wheat, sweet wheat, from which comes pancakes, pasta, toast soldiers, battered fish, butter croissants, crackers and cheese. Pulling back the canvas, I saw the grains, the color of brown rice and the shape of soup barley, realizing in that same instant that I had never before seen wheat the way it comes off the stalk. Then I smelled the urine.

"Jesus," I said. "Something's been in here."

I pulled back my hand, which I'd impulsively plunged into the kernels. As the grain resettled, I spotted the corner of a mousetrap. "Jesus," I said again.

There was a scoop inside, and, working around what proved to be a cluster of mousetraps—some of them, I thought, too large for mere mice—we began to load wheat into a tub that had until that morning held our camping gear. The stink of urine was strong, and I realized that not every grain we were scooping was in fact a grain of wheat. The pair of us fell silent, a little unnerved, a little wondering.

"Is eating wheat worth a case of hantavirus?" asked Alisa as we stepped back into the sun, arms straining under a 40-pound load.

At home I poured two cups of the Red Fife wheat berries onto a cutting board and, using my Visa card, started separating the wheat from the chaff. Outside it began to rain, a sun shower. The coast didn't need any more rain, and its arrival would only rot seeds in the ground, slow nectar flows, keep bees in the hive. It would shape the landscape, its changes, the odors and tastes of the season. There was disappointment in the rain, but also a thrill. We were sinking into this world around us, a place whose boundaries and limits we'd never really known. We now had a stake in it. Traceability had led us to this point where suddenly the rain mattered—there were beautiful red berries at stake, and the tastiest honey I'd ever put on my tongue. Distance is the enemy of awareness.

And there I sat, separating mouse shit from wheat berries with a credit card.

⇥✳ GOOSEBERRY OYSTERS ✳⇤

6 OYSTERS, CHILLED

$\frac{1}{2}$ CUP GOOSEBERRY WINE

1 HORSERADISH ROOT, PEELED AND GRATED

DRIED BULL KELP, CRUSHED

TO SHUCK THE OYSTERS, FIRMLY SLIP A KNIFE BETWEEN THE SHELL HALVES WHERE THEY MEET AT THE HINGE. TWIST UNTIL THE SHELL LOOSENS SLIGHTLY, THEN DRAW THE KNIFE AROUND THE LIP OF THE SHELL TO OPEN. POUR THE LIQUID ESSENCE INTO A BOWL AND SET ASIDE EACH OYSTER ON THE HALF-SHELL. IN A SAUCEPAN, HEAT THE WINE AND REDUCE BY ABOUT ONE-HALF AT MEDIUM BOIL. REMOVE FROM HEAT AND STIR IN THE ESSENCE. POUR A SPOON-FUL OF SAUCE OVER EACH OYSTER AND SERVE IMMEDIATELY, DRESSED WITH GRATED HORSERADISH AND A PINCH OF BULL KELP. CONSIDER: THE OYSTER IS LIKELY ALIVE WHEN YOU PUT IT IN YOUR MOUTH.

JUNE

TRULY MAN IS THE KING OF BEASTS,

FOR HIS BRUTALITY EXCEEDS THEM.

LEONARDO DA VINCI

I rounded the corner onto bustling West Fourth with a sinking feeling. Normally, the busy avenue cheers me as I slip into its flow of beautiful people with their crisp shopping bags and spa-glow faces. James and I live humbly, renters in a neighborhood we can't afford—in a city we can't afford, really. But the air is fresh and the balcony door can safely be left unlocked. Since our local-eating experiment began three months ago, however, going out to hunt for groceries had become a chore.

It was blindingly sunny, and the garage-style door of 7 Seas fish market was rolled up, opening the shop to the street. The long counter covered in glass gleamed over a bank of shaved ice heaped with ahi tuna, swordfish, sole, red snapper—the whole menagerie of the world's oceans. I examined labels for a clue to the fishes' origins, but as usual the only thing scrawled on the plastic cards were prices ranging somewhere over $10 a pound. Those sorts of prices could still shock me. I spent my teen years eating Mr. Noodles with fake crabmeat for dinner, never quite understanding that this meant we were nearly broke. It was only later I learned that my mother, widowed so young, had gone without lunches so we girls could have the thin-shaved deli meat sandwiches that would stand up to our peers' judgmental gaze. But now I was eating locally, and the beach was just eight blocks from my apartment. This would be the year of seafood.

It didn't hurt that the young man behind the counter was tall and slim with curly black hair—though he had to be sick of me. I was the irritating woman who always asked, "What do you have that's local?"

"It's almost all local," he said, gesturing widely.

I knew I could no longer trust this reply, because perceptions of what constitutes "local" vary widely. According to the Leopold Center for Sustainable Agriculture, many people wouldn't even define our 100-mile diet as "local," reserving that term for foods that have traveled less than twenty-five miles. Supermarkets have another idea entirely. To them, "local" covers a whole province or state, or even an entire country. Signs announcing "CDN/USA grown" are increasingly common in the produce department, as though we should be satisfied knowing that our food comes from somewhere within the world's second- and third-largest countries.

"What do you mean by 'local'?" I asked.

"Local in the fisheries means Alaska, B.C., Washington, Oregon. Pretty much down to California . . . Baja . . . Florida . . ."

"Not Florida!" said another clerk who was standing nearby.

"Yeah. Not Florida."

Even correcting for the Sunshine State, we were looking at a span of some 6,000 miles. As it turns out, salmon are the only fish with place-of-origin requirements, and only because of their unconsciously political life cycle: salmon may be caught in U.S. or Canadian waters, but the two nations divide their shares of the haul based on the importance of their respective salmon-spawning rivers. Shellfish, too, can be easy to trace, because they're often farmed and labeled with the precise bay they came from. As for the other fish, only better vendors such as 7 Seas had even a vague idea of where they might come from. In our part of the world, most "local" fish hailed from the Queen Charlotte Islands, an archipelago hundreds of nautical miles to the north, near Alaska. At the furthest end of the spectrum, millions of pounds of seafood taken on North America's coasts are now shipped to China to be processed—and then imported back into the United States and Canada. Dungeness crab, named for a Washington port town within our 100-mile circle, may travel 8,000 miles round trip so that Asian "crab shakers" can extract the meat. So far, the price of oil for all this transoceanic shipping has yet to close the gap between North American pay rates and the low wages of Chinese workers.

"So what's from southern B.C. or northern Washington—you know, from around here?" I asked finally.

The clerks had begun to gather and now muttered to one another. Today's salmon was from Oregon—definitely out. The octopus came from within our 100-mile radius, but I had once read that octopuses are as smart as three-year-old children, and I had never eaten them again. Finally, my young man offered,

"The snapper, the clams, or the cod." Well, I said, I'd take a fillet of cod. He weighed it and rang it up: $16.

"Hey," he said, handing me my bag, "I like your sunglasses."

All of a sudden I realized that, though there were two to four other clerks in the store at all times, he was always the one to help me. On previous visits he had explained how many pounds of mussels to serve per person (half a pound in the shell, a pound apiece for a feast), and how to shuck oysters with a butter knife. I thought of him as my personal fishmonger, a delightfully Dickensian term that helped me forget that 7 Seas is stocked with both caviar and *fleur de sel*.

"Thanks," I squeaked. I walked out the door stepping a little livelier than when I'd gone in. A bit of harmless flirting took the edge off my new role as the woman with all the questions. To those who aren't shy, it likely seems unfathomable that I could have any problem pressing people for information who are paid to provide exactly that service. I might explain by going back to my mother, who had a phobia of phoning any store or restaurant, though she did it to spare me and my sisters—who predictably developed this same aversion. And what did I do with my anxiety about meeting strangers or picking up the phone? I became a journalist. My family seems to specialize in fighting our own inclinations. My middle sister earned a degree in anthropology, which, being the study of human cultures, makes heavy interpersonal demands. She has since turned to paleobotany, the study of fossilized plants. My mother, who long said she wanted nothing more than to become a hermit, instead chose in her fifties to make a surprise transformation into a lawyer.

Life is a war of inclinations and possibilities, necessities and compulsions.

I stepped onto the balcony to test the humidity. Having lived more than half my life beside a moody ocean, I have learned that the only reliable short-term weather forecast is the feel of the air on your skin, along with certain visual clues. An exasperated weather scientist once told me, as advice for today's disconnected urbanites, "Look at the clouds. They're not just painted on the sky."

"Feels like rain," I reported to James.

"Well, then, pack a raincoat," he said. The man's stoicism could be irritating. Still, relying on the Vancouver bus system wouldn't save any time and held little appeal. I put a rolled-up jacket into my pannier and carried my bike down the stairs for the half-hour uphill journey. My set of wheels is a racing bike, state of the art circa 1986, with frayed red tape on the handlebars. James rides a ten-year-old mountain bike that aged prematurely on downhill trails. It is "raspberry" colored—bought on sale because most men apparently will not buy a pink bicycle— and has since been frankensteined with a bright blue front fork and brake cables held in place with black electrical tape. Thus do we go out in public, almost every day of the year.

In May, our Saturday-morning routine had been a trip to the farmers' market; in June it became a ride to an actual farm. Amazingly, the sixty-acre University of British Columbia Farm was a new discovery for us, despite the fact that the campus formed the western tip of the peninsula we had lived on for five years. The farm was tucked into the edge of a protected forest more than twice the size of New York's Central Park; never having been compelled to do so before, we had not sought out its odd cranny in the woods. Campus agriculture had dwindled over the late twentieth century, and the last of the farmlands had been slated for housing when a few undergraduate dreamers countered with the idea of a market garden. Today the site is the only working farm in the core of Vancouver—and home to some of the city's only chickens.

For more than fifteen years, James and I had been vegetarians. The statement came with typical caveats—we ate some wild fish, and had eaten meat while on the road in certain difficult countries. For the most part we were consistent: no meat, no eggs, no dairy. The decision was not rooted in any unusual squeamishness about killing animals. What we chose to reject was our species' capacity to disregard *life*. The cruelties are by now familiar enough: cutting off pigs' tails so they don't chew them in their depression and madness at confinement; breeding chickens with so much meatiness their legs can't support their bodies; fattening cows with industrial feed that can contain chicken and pork by-products, and even beef fat. We never will accept the idea that animals can be treated like machines that produce meat, milk, and eggs. We are equally troubled by the fact that meat production monopolizes the world's scarce agricultural land. It takes fourteen pounds of corn for a cow to gain one pound of edible meat—a fattening technique developed by industrial feedlots that goes against cows' biology; they evolved to eat only grasses. Meanwhile, cows and other livestock hog half the corn grown in America, while 800 million people go hungry worldwide. The plastic-wrapped slabs of meat in the super-market offer no clue to the animals' living conditions, so we opted out of the carnivores' world.

Until our year-long quest began, we were happily getting by on protein staples like chickpeas, lentils, dried beans, tofu, and nuts. We reveled in the fact that dinner at home often cost no more than fifty cents—and the fringe benefit that vegetarians' sweat smells less strong than meat-eaters'. So we were dismayed that we could not find any local supplier of our favorite legumes. Our vegetarian diet apparently depended on a long-distance food system heavy with environmental costs.

Now we faced the question of the chicken and the egg.

As we cycled westward through a canopy of green, the air was sweet. Rhododendron bushes were in bloom, from pale cotton candy to fuchsia, and here and there an extravagant peach. We gradually left behind the scrappy prosperity of Kitsilano—once the hippie hotbed that gave rise to Greenpeace—for the solemn wealth of Point Grey. A million dollars or more for each house, house after house, block after block. In an affordability study, Vancouver is among the English-speaking world's twenty most expensive cities, not so far below London and New York.

Not surprisingly, I had developed a real-estate obsession. I could connect it quite tidily to the seismic thirtieth birthday three years ago, as well as to the fact that, growing up, I had endured thirteen houses, six schools, and three stepfathers during a slow, 1,500-mile westward drift from the prairies where I was born. Moving had become a way of life, and, while I hated the practicalities of packing up and the strain of forever being the new kid, it also offered the possibilities of endless rebirth. My soul was always fixed on the next thing, and the next thing after that. I was never truly contented with anything—not with my work, not with our one-bedroom apartment, not even, sometimes, with James.

Like all modern-day obsessions, my mania for real estate was fueled by the internet. I wasn't only interested in what we might realistically afford, which was once a one-bedroom condo and with inflating prices had become the kind of cubicle loft that should come with a prescription for antidepressants. My scope was much broader, like that of a cuckoo that might take over any bird's nest. I applied for work in Dubai, in London, in Santa Cruz, California. I pictured myself in a charming Cape Cod saltbox, or in a discount mansion (only a few plumbing problems) in the Deep South.

Two years ago we had settled on that off-the-grid, no-road-access shack where the idea of our 100-mile diet was born. Naturally, I had found it on the internet. We flew up on a February weekend and walked in, a 26-mile round-trip through the snow along the rail line. Along the way, we had talked about hunting: if we lived in a place so remote, could we bring ourselves to live off the land? Could we shoot and butcher a moose? We had just convinced ourselves that we could—we could shoulder our rifles and kill—when we saw one. A moose, watching us from a willow thicket, close enough that we could see its eyes. Its brown, limpid, soulful eyes. We had looked at each other and laughed. By the time we made it back to our car—James had to push me gently for the final five miles, because my legs had stopped moving forward on their own—I had already made an offer in my mind for the old farmhouse perched on the Devil's

Elbow. On April Fools' Day, 2003, the twenty-three-acre river-front homestead was officially ours. I was in love with its improbability.

Inside of six weeks, I was trolling again through photographs of other homes, the supposability of other lives. It was an extension of the most powerful existential revelation of childhood: the sudden thought, perhaps while sitting in the backseat of the family car as it rolls through city streets, that every house encloses a different world, different lives, each as real as your own. Would it be possible to step through the front door and become a part of them? Was everyone else living through a tragedy—were their fathers dying, too? Or was there something somewhere out there like joy?

My bicycle wheels hummed on the asphalt. I glanced at a trim bungalow with a huge yard and thought, *$1.2 million.* If James and I had that place, Vancouver would have a second urban farm. "Everyone who eats meat should have to keep livestock," I said to James as he pedaled beside me. "But no roosters. The crowing would drive me crazy."

"You need roosters to make new chickens," said James.

Chickens were a big part of the reason we had begun riding to the UBC Farm on a regular basis. Unable to find beans and nuts, we had turned to dairy and eggs, and here at last were eggs we could eat with confidence. James, especially, made sure to check in on the chickens with every visit. Nothing was amiss. The eighty-three birds ranged in an open pasture or retired to a cozy coop. They pecked at vegetable scraps, bugs, and weeds. James had learned they were Hy-Line Browns, and even knew—more or less—their birthdays: they had all been born in December

2004. We couldn't have been more certain of their care without owning them ourselves.

There was only one problem: were they truly 100-mile chickens? I sighed as James asked the question neither of us had ever thought of before we began our experiment. The problem with animals is the feed. On the one hand, local livestock could be seen as long-distance food one step removed. On the other, the question threatened to turn ridiculous. Would we eat vegetables grown in manure from local cows that ate nonlocal feed? Would we have to ask even the vegetable farmers where their fertilizer came from? We would do our best; we would compromise. The UBC chickens were as near to a local, closed loop as we'd been able to find. Mark Bomford, program coordinator at the farm, explained that there were plans to revive grain farming on the campus. In the meantime, the cereals that supplemented the chickens' forage came in bags as the return load on a truck that delivered steel to the Canadian Prairies. It wasn't perfect, but it was striving.

We moved fast to claim a carton of eggs, all of which would be sold in the market's first hour. Such is the power of a true, golden-yellow yolk; some people show up for no other reason. Protein secured, we gathered blushing radish bunches, new potatoes, baby spinach, mixed greens, spring artichokes, and huge, yellow, summer squash blossoms. I looked forward to what James would do with the flowers: batter them with egg, and fry them.

As we tucked our harvest into packs and panniers, I caught a movement in the corner of my eye, above the crenellated line of the fir forest. I sensed an easy power. It was an eagle settling on top of the tallest tree on the clearing's edge. I had seen it exactly there the week before. From chickens to eagles: there was something deeply satisfying about these windows into the habits of other creatures.

It was the bourgeois reform movement of the late nineteenth century that banished livestock to the countryside; the campaign had been motivated in part by a proper concern for disease, but more so by obsessive tidiness. It was the poor who kept livestock, and the things that poor people did were deemed unsightly. It was yet another wedge separating people from their food. Now, a little more than 100 years later, there are signs that the barricade that keeps the farm out of the city is finally being breached. Vancouver allows backyard beekeeping again, following in the footsteps of such cities as Paris, which has an apiary on the roof of its Opera House, and Chicago, which has hives on top of City Hall. Madison, Wisconsin, and Victoria, British Columbia, have joined the list of urban areas, from London to Dallas, that permit small chicken coops.

By the time we were halfway home, I realized I was grinning. How often does that happen in modern city life? Yet all it took was this: it was Saturday morning and I had a pack full of fresh vegetables, and I was on a bicycle, and I had winked at an eagle.

James was cooking dinner while I checked the government websites that announced commercial fishery openings on the coast of British Columbia. The exercise had begun to feel pointless. There were openings often enough, but never within our 100-mile circle—never in the southern Salish Sea. The explanation was simple and sad: we had fished this area too hard and too long, and now, week in and week out, it had nothing left to give.

Tiring of reality, I turned to daydreams. Wouldn't it be lovely to live in Spain? It had been my favorite country when I did the obligatory solo backpack trip through Europe at age nineteen. Spain was hot sun and Moorish castles and paella and cheap red wine. Surely there was an affordable place somewhere in Spain.

"How do you say 'for sale' in Spanish?" I called out from where I sat. I felt a burst of impatience at the familiar sound of James chopping potatoes.

"Why?"

"I have my reasons."

"*Se vende,*" he replied, warily.

What came up in our price range was a list of *fincas,* which sounded very grand. Wasn't Hemingway's Cuban estate the Finca Vigía? The few pictures on the Spanish real-estate site showed wild and rustic hills rolling away—far away—to the sea, but the actual villas looked like homages to Stonehenge. They were the Iberian equivalent of the riverside shack we had bought in the northern forests.

"Hey," I called out, "we could start a collection of hovels around the world."

"Dinner's on," said James, trying to ignore me. He is a planner and a taker of calculated risks; freestyle daydreaming can make him so anxious he actually starts to sweat.

"I think you'd like this one," I taunted, pointing to the screen. "It used to be a sheep shed."

I sat down to a feast. I was still getting used to the vivid salads—today's was lettuce, arugula, mild radishes, and sweet kale flowers. The night's star attraction, though, was a steaming bowl of openmouthed, creamy-shelled clams and home fries, all in a garnet broth. The vegetables were from the UBC Farm and had required exactly zero fossil fuels to travel from farm to plate. The clams, I knew from the young gentleman with the dark, curly hair, were from the charmingly named Savary Island, a sandy spit of land about 90 miles north up the Strait of Georgia. The pale pink juice I couldn't identify.

"How did you cook these?" I asked, trying to sound interested rather than suspicious.

"I steamed them in the gooseberry wine," James said, "from Westham Island."

It sounded like something from *The Turnip Sandwich Cookbook*, but James seemed anxious to see me take a taste. I prized a clam from its shell and spooned it up in a pool of broth. There was a heady tang that perfectly complemented the meaty instant that the clam reached my tongue. It was a eureka moment. A total victory.

I dug into another clam and, this time, noticed a minuscule crab, the size of the nail on my baby toe. I looked into another. And found another tiny crab, frail, orange, and thoroughly steamed in wine.

They were commensal crabs, which can be found in shellfish around the world, often in great abundance in one location and hardly at all in another that might seem in every way similar. We had never seen them before, and here they were in nearly every Savary clam. The relationship between crab and clam is considered to be mutually beneficial, though no one has yet shown what the crab provides for the clam. The clam, on the other hand, offers the safest of houses. A crab will happily live its life within its confines, growing as large as the size of the clam will let it.

James was sorting his crabs from his clams, lining them up in a row along the edge of his bowl. He was playing my role, the quiet one, looking almost touched by this strange intimacy we had discovered in our soup bowls. He picked up a shell and peeped inside.

"They look comfortable," he said. A little enviously, I thought.

Our hunt for protein sources took us farther and farther afield, until an afternoon found us humming along a nowhere road aptly named Zero Avenue. I noticed an odd silver marker, then another, and I wondered aloud if they were old survey posts. "That's the American border," James said, shrugging. *That was the border?* On either side of the rural road, mirror-image Holstein cows chewed placidly in identical pastures. When we reached another metal obelisk, I asked James to stop the car. Sure enough, one side said CANADA and the other UNITED STATES OF AMERICA. I stepped one foot to the south; I was in America. The arbitrariness of history and politics was made plain in an innocent tangle of shrubbery.

The invisible line between the two nations threw a cloak of mystery over a huge section of our 100-mile circle. It was never convenient to cross a border. Even on Zero Avenue, I was beginning to see the clutter of fear and suspicion—tall poles with boxy surveillance devices on top, helicopters momentarily blocking out the sun. I hated the border guards' inane questions and the way I stammered when I answered them. But who knew what we might discover? Maybe we'd drive across and straight into a field of chickpeas. Or wheat. We still had our 40-pound tub of Red Fife from the farmer named Jim, but it was largely ignored in a corner of the living room. We had no way to grind it for flour. Boiled, the wheat berries were like chewy brown rice, but it took James an hour to separate one cup of grains from their unappetizing chaff.

We turned south into the border lineup. It's a strange passage to the other side. Vancouver has sprawled so widely now that you can drive the 35 miles to the border and never truly leave behind the suburban monster homes of the striving class. On the American side, life turns suddenly deep rural. Because the world effectively ends at the border, the people here are not a short drive from Vancouver, but rather a two-hour journey to the metropolis of Seattle. Tractors wheel along the shoulders of byways, families drive to church in all-terrain-vehicle convoys, and more than a few houses need paint.

We headed for Bellingham, population 71,000 and the seat of Whatcom County. It was a place of surprising energy, with smart cafés, boutiques, galleries, and museums filling a historic downtown core. Young men and women walked around with the same tattoos, piercings, and flannel jackets of grunge Seattle circa 1991, but here it had mellowed into something closer to the soil. We began to notice restaurants with BUY FRESH: THINK LOCAL, BE LOCAL stickers in their windows. We had apparently discovered an enlightened plane of existence; there was a year-round farm shop open seven days a week on the main street.

"Look at *these*," said James, beelining past the buckets of cut flowers and plumped rows of carrots and greens, all from the K&M Red River organic farm. He held up his cupped hands: hazelnuts.

"My god," I said, "those are almost as big as walnuts."

They were a gleaming, rich brown, like waxed teak, and larger than any I remembered from holiday nut mixes. It made sense that hazelnuts, also called filberts, would grow well here as a crop, given that the beaked hazelnut has been a favorite wild food source for the various native tribes since time immemorial. I touched a nut and felt the smoothness against my fingertips. I was sorely tempted to try one, but knew that hazelnuts could give me an uncomfortable itch in my throat and swell my lips. It was a long way back to Canada and its universal medical insurance system.

"They're only a dollar a pound," James said wonderingly. "Let's buy a huge bag."

"And take them across the border?"

"Why not?" he said. A flicker of worry passed over his features.

"You have to *declare* food products," I said. "Hazelnuts are probably illegal."

"Not if we don't declare them."

"We can't. I won't. If you want to smuggle hazelnuts, you can drop me off and I'll *walk* across the border."

"Why the hell did we come to Washington if we weren't going to bring home some food?"

It was a fair enough question. I myself couldn't really explain why the idea caused a wave of panic to pass through my body. I conjured images of border guards barking questions, cutting open seat cushions, taking James and me into separate rooms for the strip-search. I could see my name being typed into a computer, and a lifetime of delays in airports and ports of entry.

The moment's only saving grace was that we didn't have to leave the shop entirely empty-handed. The market had a detailed map of Whatcom County farms—a golden document to us, though James fumed that it wasn't much use if we were just going to stuff ourselves with what we could in the short time before returning to Canada. It got us on the move again, at least, out onto the rural routes through hamlets like Ferndale and Custer. The Nooksack River lowlands rolled in hummocks and groves, distinctly different from the Fraser Valley flats not far to the north. Neither one of us said a word when we passed a hazelnut orchard: beautiful, crooked, reaching trees with leaves so fresh they looked wet.

"The Pleasant Valley Dairy. That sounds nice," I said inanely. James must have agreed, because he started to follow the signs that took us near enough to the sea to smell the salt of Birch Bay. It was, according to our farm map, a licensed, grade-A raw-milk dairy and third-generation family farm. Certainly our first impressions were favorable. A varied herd of cattle ruminated in hock-high pasture alongside a silvery barn. Men and women in plaid climbed out of pickup trucks. Everything was human-scale; the farm store was a back room of the family house. "We're out of milk for today," called an amiable lady from behind a Dutch door as she shaved slivers of cheese for two other visitors to sample. We tried their farmstead cheese, made with a bacterial culture originally from France; a Swiss mountain variety called mutschli; and their variously seasoned goudas inspired by Holland.

"Let's get a wheel of each," James murmured, another challenge.

"That would cost a million dollars," I rejoined, not wanting to reopen the debate about crossing the border. The cheese seemed even more doubtful; I didn't think farmers were even allowed to sell raw milk in British Columbia. Maybe this cheese was actually illegal. In any case, we had plenty of artisan cheeses back home, though each cost so much that we bought them in quantities that wouldn't look out of place as bait on a mousetrap.

"How much for half a wheel of farmstead, half of apple-smoked gouda, and a chunk of mutschli?" James asked. That would be months' worth of cheese, entirely local; even the applewood for the smoking came from Whatcom County orchards.

Slowly—family farms keep their own time—the woman did the calculations. "Sixteen dollars," she said.

"Buy them," I said.

Back in the car, we made our run for the border. James would do the talking, of course. I would just try to keep my eyes off the bag that held a huge round of wrapped cheeses that we could never have afforded on our side of the border. The car smelled like applewood smoke, but the day was fine and we opened the windows.

I have to admit that I felt a little thrill as the Canadian border guard waved us onward, none the wiser.

"Damned cheese smugglers!" James shouted, shaking his fist at an imaginary international threat.

As we headed north with our booty, I thought back to that pastoral landscape, so close to home and yet subtly distinct in so many ways. In other words, a comfortable familiarity combined with the thrill of freshness—perhaps something like the feeling that once led widowed women to marry the brothers of their lost husbands. I found myself mentally settling in, somewhere along the Nooksack, standing among rows of corn, mounds of potatoes, expanses of baby greens. "Why don't we buy a place down there?" I said aloud. "We might even be able to afford it." I would wear a straw sun hat, and garden clogs, and plaid. Friends would come to visit from the north, and we would picnic in the shade of hazelnut trees, spitting apple seeds and wishing there were 100-mile lemons for lemonade. Life would be good. Life would be different.

James refused even to talk about it.

Two days before the end of June, we published our first dispatch on our progress. We put it together simply and without expectation between other deadlines, fairly certain that the outside world couldn't possibly care about some self-inflicted exile from the industrial food system. The article appeared on a vital if singularly local website called *The Tyee*, but then nothing on the internet is local. It went up at midnight, and it must have been midmorning the following day before I even thought to check up on it. There were already a dozen or so messages from readers, a strange and sudden loss of isolation. The pseudonymous "BZA" declared local eating "damn near impossible." "Peefer" worried about the conversion of farmland into housing. One writer pointed out, argumentatively it seemed, that he lived where the snow can be ten feet deep in winter, while another, who lived at the same latitude, wrote that she had wondered aloud at a seniors' home whether it was possible to eat locally in the north and was told in no uncertain terms that it was. Then there was "Lani," who knew exactly how to make jam without sugar and how to ignite the restless imagination:

> My family and I grew almost all our own food for most of my life . . . it was hard work but not that hard . . . but you do need a wee bit of land, not much, about 5 acres will do.

A wee bit of land. A new beginning.
I would bide my time.

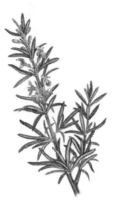

⭑ SQUASH FLOWER SOUP ⭑

1 TBSP BUTTER

1 ONION, SLICED

2 CLOVES GARLIC, MINCED

12 SQUASH FLOWERS

1 TSP SALT

$\frac{1}{4}$ TSP HOT CHILIES, GROUND

5 CUPS SEASONAL VEGETABLE STOCK

1 EGG, BEATEN

CHOP SQUASH FLOWERS, INCLUDING ANY ATTACHED STEMS. MELT BUTTER IN A LARGE SAUCEPAN ON MEDIUM HEAT. ADD ONION AND SAUTÉ UNTIL SOFT AND TURNING GOLDEN. ADD GARLIC AND FLOWERS AND COOK 2 MINUTES MORE. STIR IN SALT AND CHILIES. ADD SOUP STOCK AND BRING TO A LOW BOIL. SLOWLY POUR IN BEATEN EGG. REMOVE FROM HEAT AND COVER UNTIL EGG IS COOKED. A RECIPE FROM MEXICO CITY TO THE WORLD.

JULY

WHEN EATING FRUIT, REMEMBER WHO PLANTED THE TREE;

WHEN DRINKING CLEAR WATER, REMEMBER WHO DUG THE WELL.

VIETNAMESE PROVERB

"Getting bored yet?"

Well, yes, I am, I would say to myself. I'm getting bored with that question. It was the most common one we were asked, even as summer finally made its rightful claim to the sky. Bees, birdsong, moisture rising warm from the soil. A big farmland sun.

I might answer the question by telling people how I now liked to start the day. It wasn't with parsnip fritters anymore. Instead, I'd stumble out to the kitchen where a flat of blueberries awaited, warmed by the morning rays and burstingly ripe, thoroughly alive. Do the little fruits really, as some people claim, flush out toxins, fight cancer, plump my prostate like a pillow? I don't know, and I don't particularly care. I shoveled them into my mouth with both hands and felt like I was adding years to my life.

I might also answer by rhapsodizing about the season—and the microseasons. This early-summer harvest was ruled by the color green: lettuces, collards, mustard greens, dai gai choi and joi choi, sweet gypsy peppers, pickling cucumbers, even green tomatoes. The foodstuffs shifted week by week, but the color scheme stayed the same. The baby greens had turned big-leafed; every flavor was more robust. The slivers of snap peas were overcome by the shelling varieties, while the fava beans erupted into pods the size of sausages. Local asparagus had never appeared, but there had been fiddleheads—the tight whorls of baby ostrich ferns—and the artichoke season had been long; I have never devoured so many buttered hearts. It's worth pausing to note that many of these foods never turned up at the nearest big-box store. We were eating a more varied diet than ever before.

Or, asked the question about possible boredom, I might talk about days like the one when I walked down to the docks and met a hyperactive fisherman named Steve Johansen, one of the few who still makes his living from the Salish Sea. He's captained his own boat—the *Black Heart*—since he was twenty years old, and the young gun is still there in Johansen, hidden now behind a brush mustache, sunglasses, and the weight of more than a few years' experience. These days he's a premium independent fisherman, trusted by local restaurateurs who have begun to demand sustainable fisheries. He fishes only with trolling lines and traps, largely eliminating by-catch and damage to the seafloor.

"So what have you got today?" I asked Steve when the introductions were over.

"Spot prawns!" he said and, seeing no note of recognition in my eyes, explained that for decades British Columbia had shipped more than 90 percent of its spot prawns to Asia, where they're a delicacy, while Asia shipped tiger prawns to British Columbia. He laughed—such is life. The prawns in the hold, he said, came from rock reefs just off the Sunshine Coast, less than 50 miles away.

"I'll take two pounds," I said.

"Oh, James," he said, sticking a net into the hold, "these prawns are really small. Really small. I hope you'll like them."

Then up came the net, brimming with prawns big enough to span a dinner plate, and Steve roared with laughter as he dumped them into a case to be weighed, the prawns flicking themselves free and sending Steve chasing them across the deck. I bought 12 pounds for the freezer, the most I could afford with the money in my pocket. They were alive and venerable and what Alisa later called a perfect wedding-hat pink. Some people have a stockbroker or a drug pusher; I now had a fisherman.

The question—"Is it boring?"—is not one that people would ask about local eating in Provence or Thailand or Cajun Country, Louisiana. But places like those, where regional cuisines are treasured traditions, are a threatened minority. Ask me what dishes define the place that I live in and I will look uncomfortable and say, perhaps, "Smoked salmon." The deeper truth is that if Alisa and I had ever had anything like a "cuisine," it was the one we were inventing three meals a day in our 100-mile kitchen. Other than that, we could eat our way across North America, and increasingly the world, without really noticing that we'd left home. We eat what everyone seems to eat—but even sameness has its reasons and its history.

It wouldn't be unfair to say that Alisa and I and our several million neighbors live at the end of the world. Ours is a place of latecomers. The North Pacific coast is adequately ancient, of course, but even its indigenous peoples came at a time far advanced in the human story. Australia's Aborigines had crisscrossed their continent tens of thousands of years before even the most liberal estimate of *Homo sapiens'* arrival in the Pacific Northwest. The age of European exploration, too, found its way slowly to this ragged place; even Antarctica had been circumnavigated before a single major colonial town site was founded on the Northwest coast. By the time the European newcomers to the Salish Sea made their first effort at organized agriculture, they were caught up in a revolution in the relationship between human beings and their food. The starting point for those early settlers was an endpoint in world history.

Late July was hot in the summer of 1859. On the other side of the continent, a slavery abolitionist named John Brown was holed up in a Maryland farmhouse, planning the guerrilla raid on the federal armory at Harpers Ferry, West Virginia, that would push the United States toward civil war. In England, Charles Dickens was at the height of his literary powers, and Charles Darwin was reworking his *Origin of Species* for imminent publication. France had joined Italy in war against Austria, and here on the far rim of the newly globalized world, seventeen settlers were putting their dreams ashore at a place called Salt Spring Island, the largest of an archipelago of more than 300 islands strewn across the southern straits of the Salish Sea.

The settlers' names are lost to history, but they were likely a cross-section of their curious times. Some might have been English remittance men; others were almost certainly from among a group of more than 100 former slaves from the Zion Temple Church in San Francisco who had come north to a place unencumbered by America's slave-trading history. One, by some accounts, was "a Patagonian." Others may have been Kanakas, as Hawaiians were then known. They all had come from Victoria, where the British governor, James Douglas, had been a proper real-estate agent, sending potential colonists out for picnics to a Salt Spring landing called Walker Hook. Douglas was eager to build his agricultural capacity—the population of Victoria was booming with gold-rush hopefuls, but the immense North Pacific landscape remained a comfortable home only to natives and trappers, and its boundaries were lawless and contested. On the same day that Salt Spring was colonized, twenty-five miles due south on disputed San Juan Island an American military unit would land in a game of international brinksmanship that began, absurdly, when a British pig was shot in a Yankee potato patch. It would take thirteen years to confirm San Juan as American soil.

Walker Hook is the kind of place that real-estate agents still use to make impulse sales. It is a tidy harbor, a snug protected by a spine of forest and rock that declines at the bay's head into a long curve of eelgrass and sand. In the sun the hook flares white—the beach is a midden, one of the thousands of places where the Coast Salish people had feasted on clams, oysters, and mussels and left the shells to be ground smooth by the tides. Despite decimation by the plagues that had traveled up the coast well ahead of the European galleons, the Salish remained ubiquitous on the shores of their namesake sea, and the Salt Spring settlers arrived in a Salish canoe, a high-prowed boat well designed for the Pacific's inside channels. That night, according to island storytellers, one of the Zion Temple congregation stood at the campfire and said, "We are a free people! This is our island!" Then he broke into song.

What all this history is drifting toward is a handful of truths, the kind that shape a place at its roots and refract all that has come before and since. One might fruitfully compare the Salt Spring settlers to the colonists who landed near the abandoned Wampanoag Indian village of Patuxet in 1620. The renowned New Plymouth settlement of English religious separatists, who would go on to be known as the Pilgrims and inspire the Thanksgiving tradition, was immediately shaped by the land they encountered, and its people. Arriving in November, the colonists survived their first winter by raiding the stored supplies of the Wampanoag, whose population had been devastated by European diseases. Of the 101 English who came ashore, fifty-two survived to the harvest feast in 1621. The colonists had been aided, in an act of almost unbelievable generosity, by a Wampanoag translator named Tisquantum (better known by his bastardized name, Squanto), who was one of the few survivors of the Patuxet plagues and who had learned English after being kidnapped and put on show in Europe. With a diplomatic agreement in place that the settlers and the Wampanoag would defend each other from military assaults, Tisquantum showed the colonists how to raise corn and fertilize their fields with fish. Most of what is known of their "first Thanksgiving" comes from a single, 115-

word paragraph in a letter written by one of the settlers. Possible menu items are believed by scholars to have been limited to corn raised from Wampanoag seed, and five deer provided by the ninety visiting Wampanoag warriors, plus wild turkeys and other fowl, fish and shellfish, wild nuts and berries, and a local species of squash.

Two hundred thirty-nine years later, the Salt Spring pioneers hardly paused to consider the staple foods of the Salish and other coastal tribes. Had they done so, Alisa and I might have had an alternative to three meals a day of 100-mile potatoes. We might have been "flower eaters," roasting the common camas bulbs that were so carefully tended by the Salish that the first British captain to see Vancouver Island was reminded of the English gardens of home. Farther south, the American explorer Meriwether Lewis witnessed the purple-blue camas in fields so large and dense with blossoms that he mistook them for "lakes of fine clear water." We might have been people of flowers and salmon and berries, with treasured pots of oolichan grease, a fermented paste of North Pacific smelt that was among the most valuable trade items on the coast before the arrival of the European invaders. We might at least have contented our sweet tooths with the unique soapberry froth remembered as "Indian ice cream."

Instead, our forebears simply and immediately began to re-create the food culture of Europe. They unloaded their sacks of seeds, their laying hens, their apple-tree sprigs that were packed in potatoes to nourish the rootstocks through months of being shipped in the bellies of tall ships. The New World cultures had given Europe tomatoes, chilies, potatoes, corn, squashes, vanilla, sunflowers, chocolate—the list goes on and on. But by the time the world-beating colonials reached their farthest frontiers, they no longer needed or cared for indigenous foods. There would be no northwestern equivalent to succotash. Nor would there be time for the new settlements to develop anything as distinctive as, for example, *cramaillotte,* the wild dandelion-flower jelly made by a single specialist in a single village in France. The first truly global food system was in action, and only one foodstuff would ever become synonymous with the vast and verdant Pacific Northwest: smoked salmon. It took the continent by storm in the late nineteenth century—just as soon as Pacific salmon could be sent by rail to be smoked in Manhattan.

Not quite 150 years later, Dan Jason and I stood in Salt Spring's high Blackburn Valley, surrounded by various Hindu deities and tranquillity fountains, none of which is precisely Dan's cup of tea. The land he works helps feed a yoga center, but Dan Jason's natural mystic is the humble seed. He worships at the altar of variety.

"You see back there? That's the bean field. There's—well, I cut down a bit this year. There's about eighty varieties back there." Dan was trying to distract me so that he could finish the job he was working on when I arrived, right about when I said I would, which is not the way time typically works on the Gulf Islands. I wandered off to suss out the beans, and Dan dropped back onto his hands and knees, his bare feet as dusty as an apostle's, to continue tamping the roots of tomato seedings into the soil.

All of Dan's fields are variations on the same pattern: long rows of plants that, with a few exceptions, all look *almost* the same. Even the untrained eye, though, picks up a jigsaw puzzle of subtle differences, a paint-chip shading of greens from Amazon to jade to Kelly to Celtic to reef to emerald to Miami. I studied the wooden markers at the head of each row, losing myself in the names of beans. Cannellini, Lake Kivu Pearls, Sangre de Toro, Moroccan chickpea, Cheetah, Leopard, Black Coco, Aztec red kidney, Stevenson Blue Eye, Gnuttle Amish, Shirofune soybean, Big Mama, Rojo de Seda, Dr. Wynche's, Molasses Face, Orca. One, called Ruckle, is a Salt Spring breed that dates back nearly to Walker Hook. I wandered back to where Dan was now finished with the tomatoes (he grew an incredible 300 varieties in 2005) and took a downwind whiff of some forty types of garlic. Dragging hoses across a field, Dan explained that he introduces about eighty new varieties of seed each year.

"Where do you get them?" I asked.

"Often, sadly enough, it's from farms that are closing down. People will say, 'Can you please keep this growing? Because it's been in our family for eighty years and my aunt used to love this kind of bean.' Things like that."

Salt Spring is a microcosm. All across the island the farmscape is fading. It is possible to stand in Dan Jason's fields and look out on a pattern of loss that stretches the breadth of North America. On the other hand, taking the near view, we can see how the melancholy process affects one given place. And we can name names.

J.R. Anderson was a colonial bureaucrat, which makes it tempting to imagine him as a frontier paper-pusher, more concerned with cricket scores sent from London than with the lives of pioneer farmers. That assumption would miss the mark. The

Anderson family's interest in the Americas reached back at least as far as J.R.'s great-grandfather, who corresponded chummily with George Washington, though it was J.R.'s father who went west, inspired by the adventure novels of James Fenimore Cooper. Little J.R. was born in 1841 at Fort Nisqually, in what is now Washington State. It was not a soft life. When, at age nine, J.R. was finally sent to school, it was by horse pack train over mountain passes, then by boat down the Fraser, and finally by seagoing Salish canoe, the wide gulf of the Strait of Georgia reminding him of the painful absence of his father. The final crossing to Victoria by night was imprinted on his mind: the "terror of the rough sea" and "the savage crew and their terrifying canoe songs," each paddle stroke lit by the eerie green glow of phosphorescent plankton. His new home was essentially three muddy roadways. It was a place where young boys had to weed the school garden until they could sneak off to tie blocks of wood to dogfish tails and laugh as the fish tried to dive. J.R. ate his first apple in Victoria, and disliked it.

In 1891, Anderson was appointed to oversee agriculture in the province of British Columbia. "I found absolutely nothing had been done," he would write in his unpublished memoirs, "not the scratch of a pen, no books nor papers to guide me." What he found, through surveys and excursions, was a network of farms that resided somewhere between self-sufficient local production and commercial growing for a wider market. It was a farming culture that, to him, looked like the past, and to a person today might look something like the future.

Consider Salt Spring Island in 1893. It was a bum year, with a "cold backward spring" and a sodden summer and autumn. Nonetheless, the island, just seven by sixteen miles and home to only ninety people, produced 74 tons of peas, 156 tons of potatoes, 185 tons of miscellaneous root crops, 121,000 pounds of fruit, 2,210 pounds of butter, 4,500 pounds of wool, and 6,305 dozen eggs. There were families living on much smaller islands who were totally self-sufficient; Salt Spring had food to spare. Even the year's apple harvest, considered "almost a total failure," could have provided seven apples a day to every islander; the more successful potato crop could have supplied even the current 10,000 Salt Spring residents with a 125-pound bag of spuds for every family of four.

Even these figures fail to measure the wealth of the early farming communities. There was also an incredible genetic diversity. Salt Spring was famous for apples. Of the varieties grown there in 1893 alone, there is only one that I have ever tasted: Gravenstein. That leaves me ignorant of the following: Wealthy, Northern Spy, Baldwin, Canada Reinette, Blenheim Orange, Red Astrachan, Gloria Mundi, Yellow Belle Fleur, Haas, Duchess of Oldenburg, Ben Davis, Golden Russett, Fallawater, Golden Noble, Alexander, Rhode Island Greening, King of Tompkins County, Fameuse, Dunclow's Seedling, Lord Derby, King of Pippins, Warner's King, Irish Peach, Early Harvest, Roxbury Russet, Blue Pearmain, Hubardson's Nonsuch, Maiden's Blush, and Winter Bellfleur. A popular local poem comes to mind: the title is "Say the Names."

And there was wheat. Oh, how there was wheat, and barley, and oats, 251 acres of them on Salt Spring alone, producing 144 tons of grain even in that lousy year. Dozens of strains could be found within 100 miles of the place where Alisa's and my apartment block stands today. Red Fife was popular, but every township had its microclimate and a wheat seed to go with it. Say the names: 90-day, White Fife, Chili, Club, Ladoga, Spring Swamp. Wheat was growing everywhere. Pancakes, biscuits, gravy, sourdough, Yorkshire pudding, everywhere. Up the Fraser Valley in Agassiz, the Dominion Experimental Farm had, one year earlier, crossed three varieties to create a new breed called Marquis. No one knew it then, but it was the dawn of modern monoculture. By World War I, Marquis wheat would account for almost 50 percent of all wheat grown in the United States and 80 percent in Canada. At its peak of popularity, Marquis waved over more than 20 million acres of North America, before passing on its genes to newer crop cultivars with names like today's Proven 5602HR.

J.R. Anderson saw it coming. He could feel the bearing toward industrialization, economic specialization, a global market that was brought closer with every new stretch of road and rail. "There is no doubt in my mind," he wrote in his annual report, "that if the farmers would confine themselves principally to dairying, fruit culture, and root crops in the Lower Country, leaving cereals to those of the Upper Country, it would result much more favorably to the interests of all."

A century later, the process that J.R. Anderson had predicted, and which had already engulfed much of the Western world, was reaching its eventual conclusion. I was one of its products, a person who had lost so much history and knowledge that I could believe that wheat could not be grown where I live. Dan Jason had once been the same. "I started exploring the beans and chickpeas, and grains, kamut and quinoa—and they all worked. I was just so amazed," he told me. He didn't learn until much later that the field he was planting had, in 1890, given a harvest of Red Fife wheat.

The grand experiment in industrial agriculture had its successes, and only a fool would try to argue otherwise. The daily food supply in America now contains enough calories to feed almost double the U.S. population, without reducing food exports by one iota. People spend 7 percent of their disposable income on food, down from 22 percent in 1950. A European farmer prior to World War II fed an average of five people; a single American farmer today feeds twenty-five times as many. But the system has also had its colossal failures and losses. Arguably the greatest among these was the undoing of the local, of specific experience and autochthonous knowledge. One can list peculiar and particular outcomes, like the extinction of 436 out of the 463 varieties of radish that were known to the U.S. Department of Agriculture in the early twentieth century. Or the fact that 80 percent of the yearly tomato crop in the United States is harvested while it's still green. Or the fact that Salt Spring Island today produces just 2 percent of its residents' food.

History is turning back toward the small with new intelligence and purpose. Dan Jason now sells seeds to 6,000 people each year; in return, his collection is only increasing. Three years ago he received a packet of seeds that had been found in a carbon-dated urn uncovered at a native burial site near the Great Lakes. His 1,000-Year Tobacco grows fine in his fields, just as tobacco did for settlers more than a century ago, when I would have been able to buy a 100-mile cigar. We're moving backward *and* forward, Dan explained. There are now, by his estimate, 375 varieties of apple grown on Salt Spring Island, possibly more than at any point in its history.

I had one more question for him: "What's something that surprised you? What's something that you never thought would turn out, and then did?"

Dan's fingers worked the soil around two mystery sprouts, one from South Africa and one from Zimbabwe. Finally he turned to me. "I can't really think of anything."

"You've never planted anything that didn't work out?"

"No," he said. "I've just never thought they wouldn't."

In the end, Dan Jason could not lead us to wheat. One hundred fifty people had bought his Red Fife seeds that year, but the only local growers he knew had nothing but trial batches. Not even the hive-mind of the internet, through which the 100-mile diet had now touched down in Norway, France, and Australia, could Google us up some good local flour.

It was an internet tip, however, that led us off in search of farmgate goodies just off a stretch of suburban highway. Nothing about the journey made sense: not the dense flow of traffic, the plaster crush of houses, the white noise that filled the valley. Then I saw the sign at a side road:

ORGANIC BLUEBERRIES $2/LB

"Jesus, James, you'll get us killed!" shouted Alisa as I hit the gravel shoulder and swung into a U-turn.

I brake for blueberries.

The road was a typical cul-de-sac. Pulling in at the signposted driveway, though, we could see acreage—not a lot, but enough, and every inch of it in use. The now-familiar blueberry bushes filled a field behind a windbreak hedge. We got out of the car.

"Hel-lo," said a woman's voice with the careful pronunciation of English as a foreign language. We turned to see a slim, conservatively dressed woman. "You want blueberries?"

"Can we see?" said Alisa, gesturing to the field not 20 feet away.

"Come," said the woman.

We walked together to the bushes, our guide running a hand through the leaves. "You see, there are beautiful berries. The smell, beautiful," she said, and we nodded. There wasn't much to say, so we just stood there, breathing, in an urban oasis. Walking back, I spotted a long trellis arch. There were grapes there, and the woman led us to them, stripped off two clusters, one purple and one green, and handed them to us. "Please, eat," she said. They were impossibly sweet. And then, among the vines, I saw something else, a collection of pendulous, tromboning vegetables, some almost as tall as me. They were a variegated yellow-green, and looked like something that would slice cool and moist under the day's hot sun. "And what are those?" I asked.

"What?"

"Those. Can I buy one?"

"Those are for tempo," she said.

"Tempo?"

"You know, like Buddha tempo."

"Buddhist temple!"

"Yes, Buddha temple. All for temple. Not for sale."

"I can't buy one?" I tried to look charming, and maybe even a little bit Buddhist. She shook her head, apologetic but firm.

"What is it called?" I asked, still reluctant to leave a new foodstuff behind. "What is its name?"

"Its name?" she asked, looking at me quizzically. *"Wach,"* she said.

"Wach," I tried. I could see, now, that the plaster house contained, in what might once have been a garage, a simple Vietnamese Buddhist temple. I was fascinated: a farm-slash-temple, where the faithful gathered to carve the *wach,* which must not be sold to just any Caucasian who swaggered up with his pocket full of change. We sampled the berries, which made up for their small size with a concentrated flavor that left my mouth with a perfumed taste. We bought a ten-pound flat of them, and it wasn't until we were well down the road that I realized I was an idiot. It wasn't *wach* that the woman was saying, but *squash,* apparently of a variety much loved in Vietnam but previously unknown to me here.

And this was the lesson of the suburban farms that we discovered that day. Just a few blocks from the sacred squash were the Chinese market gardens of Fook Shing Farm, where we bought fuzzy melons, Chinese cabbages, Asian radishes, chois, watercress, and a bitter courgette called *mo qua.* Not far away, the descendents of farmers from India sowed coriander and *knolkhol* (a kind of kohlrabi). At the UBC farm, we knew, visiting Mayan gardeners were succeeding with amaranth, Andean potatoes, and a green called *yerba mora.* There is no manifest destiny in the foods that most of us think of as "local." They are cultural artifacts, the result of politics and market trends and demographics. We have only begun to sow what we might reap.

With star fruit and durian now available at the megamart, it is easy to believe that turbo-capitalist globalization is the best—perhaps the only—way to diversify what we put on our plates. In reality, those same forces have tended to diminish our collective food culture. Not only have we forgotten much of what our landscapes once produced; we have never known the full range of possible crops. According to the biologist and author Edward O. Wilson, some 7,000 species of plant are known to have been used by different human societies throughout history. Today, just twenty species provide 90 percent of the world's food. In *The Diversity of Life,* Wilson points to fruit as the best illustration of a "pattern of underutilization." About a dozen familiar fruit species dominate the northern market and have been heavily adopted in tropical regions as well. Meanwhile, some 200 additional species are currently cultivated or collected in the tropics, and at least 3,000 others are waiting to be put into use. All told, at least 30,000 plant species are known to have edible parts.

Suddenly the well-stocked aisles of my local globalized grocery don't seem such a horn of plenty. Will we ever have mass markets for 30,000 plant foods? It's unlikely, if not impossible. That degree of variety only makes sense at a small scale, at the intimate levels of community and place. This we can say for certain: it is anything but boring.

Toward the end of July, a work trip took me for a day to Victoria, where the year's last camas flowers bloomed in the city parks that were once Salish meadows. I found myself driving to the outskirts of town, winding along old roads that I remembered from my student years. I used to do this sort of thing: wander the countryside, usually with a brace of field guides, with stops to identify wildflowers or mushrooms or birds. There was a time when I had more time.

Finally I found what I was looking for and pulled over. A forest meadow climbed overhead, shaded here and there by the Halloween shadows of Garry oaks. It was a perfect place to find camas, and I did, the dark purple flowers already shedding petals. The meadow death-camas was here, too, I noted. With its cream-colored blossoms beginning to wither, it could easily be mistaken for its cousin. As the name suggests, the death-camas bulb is lethally poisonous. I would need to choose carefully.

I started digging. The camas stems plunged into the earth, and it was harder work than I'd expected. I clawed my way down until the dirt was almost gravel, until blood creased the edge of one fingernail. There it was, at last, the bulb. It was a large one, roughly the shape and size of a head of garlic; I was lucky. Moving on, far from the first, I dug for a second. It was small and shallow, and I left it in place, then rooted once more, down, down, prying aside a stone to uncover the quarry. It was a potent act, this digging. Besides being an agricultural bureaucrat, J.R. Anderson had been a botanist and a clear-eyed observer of his world. In 1929, one year before a driver ran him down at the age of eighty-nine, he had published a guide to the food, medicinal, and poisonous plants of this region. The book is a precious thing, full of knowledge and scenes that are no more. How a bough from an ocean spray shrub can make a trusty fishing rod. How local markets once sold heaps of wild shotberry, one of the only native plant foods to enjoy a few forgotten years of popularity. Anderson's tender description of the gathering and preparation of camas bulbs convinced me that he had done exactly this, searched the earth for the tranquil corm. Meanwhile, unbeknownst to me, the Lekwungen Salish, descendents of the original residents of the area, had, on June 22, 2005, held their first camas harvest in 150 years.

I came home with my two bulbs, feeling very much the successful provider. It was an otherwise typical day for Alisa and me: the refrigerator had become a menagerie of the unexpected. There might be radishes, *yerba mora,* sage, clams, the Red Fife wheat berries, and *mo qua.* I would plumb recipe books, search the internet, transform old standbys, but everything, now, was at its essence terra incognita. And isn't that how cookeries as distinct as those of Tuscany and Provence, not to mention the Coast Salish, evolved? Innovation moves at the speed of necessity.

I wanted to taste the camas simply, however. I roasted the bulbs in tinfoil, long and slow, hoping to replicate something like an earthen cooking pit. They came out soft, with a texture like roasted garlic but with brighter white flesh. I called Alisa to the table and we ate, with no more ritual than an unusual silence. The bulbs were a bit sweet, a bit gummy, with a nuttiness like sunchokes. Only the most distant aftertaste was faintly floral. Really, they were a bit bland. Imagine trying to describe the taste of a potato to someone who'd never eaten one.

We felt like pioneers setting foot on a strange place called home.

⇢⚜ BRAISED DANDELION GREENS ⚜⇠ WITH MORELS

BUTTER

5 CLOVES GARLIC, MINCED

1 LB DANDELION GREENS

1 LB MOREL MUSHROOMS

SALT

RED CHILIES, GROUND

SELECT THE YOUNGEST DANDELION GREENS FROM PLANTS THAT HAVE NOT FLOWERED (SWEETEST IN SPRING, WITH A HARD EDGE MIDSEASON, SWEETER AGAIN AFTER FROST). SOAK FOR SEVERAL HOURS IN PLENTY OF COLD WATER TO REDUCE BITTERNESS. AT THE SAME TIME, SOAK THE MORELS IN SALTED WATER TO CLEAN AND, IF THE MUSHROOMS ARE DRIED, TO REHYDRATE. HEAT 1 TBSP BUTTER IN A CAST-IRON SKILLET. SAUTÉ GARLIC FOR 2 MINUTES. DRAIN MUSHROOMS, SLICE, AND SAUTÉ UNTIL THEY RELEASE THEIR JUICES. SET SAUTÉED MIXTURE ASIDE IN A BOWL. ADD 1 TBSP BUTTER TO SKILLET AND HEAT TO MEDIUM-HIGH. DRAIN BUT DO NOT DRY GREENS AND CHOP INTO 3-INCH PIECES. ADD TO SKILLET AND COVER. WHEN GREENS HAVE WILTED AND JUST BEGUN TO BLACKEN, REDUCE HEAT, ADD MUSHROOM-AND-GARLIC BLEND, AND SAUTÉ 1 MINUTE MORE. SERVE BY THE LIGHT OF EMERGENCY CANDLES.

AUGUST

When we left Vancouver in the first days of August, a yellow smog hung over the Fraser Valley, and smoked wild salmon was going for thirty-five dollars a pound. Good-bye to all that; we were driving north to Dorreen. Because it takes two days to get there, we planned to stay for a month—and in that time we would not turn on a light, use a refrigerator, drive a car, ride a bus, have a hot shower, or even return the e-mails of fellow local-food enthusiasts. Not until the day we returned to "civilization."

To reach Dorreen, you drive to Terrace, which rhymes with Paris, and so we had nicknamed it the Paris of the North. It should be that: if it were in Europe there would be a bustling plaza from which to admire the wide bowl of surrounding mountains. If it were in America it would be legendary, every steelhead and king salmon stream immortalized by Norman Maclean and Woody Guthrie. But this is northern Canada, and so, on the riverfront, there is simply a Wal-Mart.

The drive to Terrace is made unnecessarily long, sixteen hours, by the wonderful fact that the landscape is not riven with highways. There is no direct route up the British Columbia coast. You have to drive eastward, over the mountains beyond the town of Hope, then north through the dusty Cariboo ranch country that thickens into the boreal forest. To this point, the route roughly follows the Fraser River, but then you hook westward again, back to the Coast Mountains, the same range that encloses Vancouver. Lost among those peaks, you finally stumble upon the Skeena, "River of Mists," and by the time it opens into the alluvial plain at Terrace, you are only 200 feet above sea level. Here you are cheek-by-jowl with the southern tip of Alaska, the trees grow giant again, and every town has at least one totem pole. This is the rain-forest territory of the Kermode—the pure white bear that environmentalists have christened the spirit bear. We haven't seen one around Dorreen, but Dolsa, the forty-something woman who is the only year-round resident of the place, has. It was drunk, she said. A train carrying wheat derailed outside of Dorreen, and the grain began to ferment in the summer heat. Then along came the spirit bear, who proceeded to get spirited indeed.

To be honest, we had thought that our summer break in Dorreen would also be an unavoidable holiday from local eating. This was latitude 55 degrees north, among mountains that wear garlands of glaciers.

"Was that a farmers' market?" I said to James.

"What?"

"Turn around," I said. James, like many men, hates to stop

when he is in travel mode. Backtracking would require the firm tone that I otherwise reserve for making him go to the doctor.

"What? I didn't see anything."

"Turn. Around."

We were in the town of Smithers, population 8,000 and the last stop before Terrace, and sure enough the good citizens— Smithereens?—were lining up in front of stalls. There was only a cluster of booths, but each was overflowing with the bounty you would find at more southerly markets: lettuce, cucumbers, carrots, potatoes, squash, beans, basil, and more. Everything on sale seemed to be the largest I had ever seen. "We get nineteen hours of daylight this time of year," shrugged a farmer when I asked. James came bobbing toward me, grinning, with a cabbage on his shoulder that was bigger than his head. We needed vegetables like these, foods that could survive without refrigeration for two weeks or more. We were back to shopping for war vegetables.

An old man sat completely still behind a hand-lettered sign: WILLY'S. All he had for sale were tomatoes. Nothing is more delicate, and therefore less Dorreen-friendly, than a ripe garden tomato, which stands in stark contrast to the tough commercial varieties that are bred to survive transcontinental travel. But old Willy was all alone. I moved toward him, ignoring James as he gestured to stop me. He had already seen, I suppose, that the tomatoes were unpromisingly small, with a worrisome yellow streaking like anemic tiger stripes. But I was in it now. Old Willy was smiling at me; I had gotten his hopes up. It wasn't like I could settle on some other item, because all he had were these runt tomatoes. Willy drew out the process of settling them into a bag and handing me my change, though he spoke not a word. Back where James was standing, I held open the bag for him to see inside, and tried to look contrite.

"I knew they wouldn't be any good," he harrumphed.

I was still cradling my fragile cargo in my arms as we stepped onto the train that is the last leg of the journey to Dorreen. The conductor greeted us warmly; the crew always remembers us from year to year. It is touching, the way that railroad work still seems to be so much more than just a job. Dorreen is a favorite place along this, the Skeena Line from the coast at Prince Rupert to the Rocky Mountain hamlet of Jasper; along with its beauty, the workers appreciate that the lone, sort-of-inhabited town is still rail-dependent.

The fifteen-dollar ride from Terrace is a scenic wonder, the tracks bracketed by the wide, rushing Skeena and summit alpenglow. Soon we passed through the choking rapids of Kitselas Canyon, where in ancient times a toll was charged to pass between the territories of the Tsimshian and Gitksan Indians. We passed through the oddball town of Usk, connected to the world by an auto ferry in the warm months and a gondola through the winter. "This is one of only two remaining 'reaction' ferries in British Columbia," the conductor spoke into her loudspeaker for the benefit of the tourists, who filled most of the seats in the two passenger cars. "It's powered by the river current alone."

James was carving a tomato into quarters to pass the time. We popped them into our mouths. I took James's expression for a mirror of my own.

"Old Willy didn't let us down," he said.

They burst in the mouth, with a sweet, warm juice. These were tomatoes picked the moment they were ripe, perfectly ripe, the kind of tomato the Queen would receive at teatime, on toast, and believe that the Empire was still capable of great things. Willy and I hadn't exchanged a single word, but he would be fixed in memory, a part of my map of the world: I already knew that we would be back, probably a year from now, to look for more of his tomatoes.

"Coming up is the ghost town of Dorreen," the conductor announced. "Look in the window of the general store and you'll see one of the residents." The train slowed past the peeling clapboard station, and the tourists could be heard tittering as they spotted the mannequin that some wag had propped up, waving, in the second story of a store that hadn't stocked anything for forty years. "Two more are on the train right now," she continued, *"city slickers gone country."* She said these words kindly, but necks were craning all through the car for a look at the fools who were, surely, some reverse of the Beverly Hillbillies. I looked stonily ahead, my cheeks pink, as we walked the long aisle to the door. Standing railside as the baggage man handed down our gear, I blinked to the irritating flash of cameras from the first-class dome car.

But who could blame the shutterbugs? Dorreen may well be the best-tended ghost town in the world. There is a ramshackle row of early 1900s houses, with the quirky general store at the center of a large rectangular clearing walled in by evergreens. An occasional summer resident named Ed, from California, keeps the clearing tidy with a ride-on mower he brought in god knows how. Dolsa, dubbed The Mayor, makes continual rounds on her all-terrain vehicle, a water canteen slung over her shoulder, to ensure that the old trails stay clear and all is well in the peaceable kingdom.

The sound of the train faded into the distance, and the overwhelming silence rushed in. For the next thirty days, James and I would be without friends, family, movie theaters, shops, a radio, or even a telephone. The thought caused me some anxiety. Already it could be hard to find something new to say across the breakfast table.

At the front porch of the general store, we stopped to check the logbook, in which everyone but Dolsa leaves comments. The most recent entry, from a week before, talked of picking cherries in the orchard. The orchard was ours, but we were glad that the fruit was being used. I thought eagerly of the cherry-ade I had invented the previous year. Though technically sour cherries, the Dorreen variety is sweet enough to eat plain off the tree; each is a jewel, with a red translucent skin made impossibly bright by the sun. They are juicy, perfect for pies, and I have never seen anything remotely like them in a supermarket. The first trees had been planted perhaps eighty years ago; in fact, the whole orchard was a living library of old-fashioned fruits. Ed, an apple enthusiast, took a couple of cuttings home to California to graft onto his own trees. He prized the resulting fruit so much that he took one to an apple institute, which declared it a Shenandoah Strawberry. I once punched the name into Google: nothing. These old varieties are not the kind of information that is of interest to the Information Age; they make themselves known only when you stand in front of them. When ripe, the Shenandoah Strawberry is a beautiful two-tone of green blushing to the pink side of red. It's an eating apple, crisply white-fleshed, while the harvest of our two other trees are best for sauce. Then there are the twin crab apples and a plum.

Our cabin is fifteen minutes from the railbed, a peaceful promenade down a trail through the pine forest. At a curve in the road, we often see a grouse. If it is early in the season and she is with her chicks, she sometimes attacks—a display that is both comical and terrifying. By the time we can hear the grumble of the Devil's Elbow rapids, we are among soaring poplars. The trees sway steeply in high wind, ship masts in a storm, with a noise that is sometimes like old men grumbling around a table, and other times like ghostly singing. Finally the trail opens into a thimbleberry grove where we often see a resting toad. In one spot near here I saw a slug—I repeat, a *slug*—perform a leap from one leaf to another, leading me to wonder what we may not yet know of the secret lives of humble creatures.

For half of the last century, our riverside property was a working farm, shipping produce by train the 125 miles to coastal Prince Rupert. Starting in the 1950s, Dorreen became a part of that great receding tide of things local and small-scale. The trains came less often, the farms went fallow, the general store closed, and, in a final stroke, the town lost its lone phone booth in the 1980s. Our house, too (and here I have to admit to the temptation to put everything about Dorreen in quotation marks: "house," "store," "town"), has been so long abandoned that it has become habitat. There are bats and squirrels and mice in the walls, a weasel in the woodpile, and the space beneath the floorboards is an occasional summer home for a porcupine. The butterflies, meanwhile, have come to regard the house as their preserve.

When we first open the door, they drift in all day long. Within a few days, by whatever means butterflies use to pass on messages, they decide to stay outside. They rest on the westward wall, gently fanning their wings in the afternoon sun.

It is hard to overstate the building's complete dilapidation. The local tax assessor lists its value as zero dollars. The walls, originally painted a cheerful yellow, are now a brittlewood gray. The tin roof has been rippled by ten thousand windstorms, and several of the windows are covered with plastic sheeting. Only the new woodstove chimney, installed by James last summer at a cost of dozens of hammer blows to his thumb, rises silver and shining above the sorry scene.

I was surprised to see that the cherry tree limbs were bare. "Looks like the cherries are over for the year," I said. Then we saw that branches were snapped off at the joints, the breaks ragged and raw.

"A bear ate them all," James said.

I peered through a squirrel hole directly into the cabin's kitchen and foresaw a lot of long nights ahead.

Not too many days ever pass in Dorreen without a trip to Fiddler Creek. The trail is another sun-kissed old road, perfect for hand-holding. After not even two miles, the path opens onto the train tracks and a railway bridge with a view of heaven. Framed by a glaciated cirque of fantastical mountains, the creek leaps its way to the bottom and rushes beneath your feet. Turning, you can see where its blue-green water swirls into the muddy summer freshet of the Skeena. Dolly Varden lurk in the deeper pools.

Visitors often spend hours fishing this confluence, almost as often without luck. Once, though, we saw a Gitksan fisherman wade in up to his knees with only a hook on a hand line, and catch three Dollies inside of twenty minutes. Almost anywhere else, Fiddler Creek would be a river; here it is a creek in comparison to the churning Skeena. This is not a gentle land: everything is fast and cold and steep and rocky and utterly grand.

The creek mouth is an old Gitksan reserve that no one has lived on for years. Like everyone else, the Gitksan shifted to the other side of the Skeena when the road was built there to move American troops to the Pacific during World War II. The towns on the rail side of the river, like Dorreen, began their long decline. Today their isolation has become their attraction. The Gitksan have been slowly building an eco-tourism camp alongside the creek. We walked among the silent heavy machinery, the half-finished buildings that were waiting for new funding. It took a moment to register that there was a man in the forest looking out at us. An animal instant passed, wordless, a primal rush of curiosity and fear. Then a black-and-white collie mutt rushed toward us, barking and snarling. The man didn't call off the dog.

"Hello, Roy," said James, with the emphatic cool that lets me know he is as uncertain about a situation as I am.

So it was Roy. We had only met him once, last summer, in passing. He had seemed friendly enough, and his dog had been a different creature then, outside of his home territory and therefore submissive. There were those, though, who were a little afraid of Roy. The Gitksan had taken him on as guardian of Fiddler

Creek, and it was a job he took seriously. He is a person who lives year-round in the bush, and that is enough to raise a yellow caution flag for almost anyone else.

"James and Alisa, come on up," he said, amazing me with his memory. Roy is not tall, but he is the wiriest man I expect to meet in my lifetime, all taut tendons and striated muscle. It would be hard to say that he seemed to relax, but he bustled around, eager to make us feel at home in the circle of tamped earth outside his canvas caravan tent. He introduced us to his teenaged son, visiting from the outside world. They had been preparing for a serious day of fishing, but Roy put down the stick he was whittling for a gaff and rushed inside the dark confines of the tent to bring out a ripped vinyl dinette chair, his best for the lady guest. We made small talk around a low fire; the day was hot, but a fire is a good companion. James wandered off into the forest with Roy's son to shoot a .22 at a plastic bottle and came back smiling, having nailed it on the second shot. Score one for the city slickers.

"This calls for a celebration," said Roy. He ducked again into the tent, emerging this time with an unmarked bottle of liquid as clear as the Virgin Mary's tears. He passed the bottle around, and when it came to me I took not a sip, but the requisite swig. Instantly, I felt a part of my brain die. It was moonshine, sweet and harsh and tasting faintly of potatoes. The light of the afternoon seemed to lengthen.

Soon, Roy was in a storytelling mood. Yes, he had been in the bush for many years, but not always the *same* bush. He had logging stories and mushroom-picking stories. In the Cariboo Mountains, he said with some pride, he and a friend had been the first two people ever thrown into a town's new jail. Discovering that we had a black bear in our part of the woods, he made the gentlemanly offer of a bearskin vest and a share of the meat, which he would smoke; we hinted that we preferred to let the bear wear the vest for now. He didn't seem to understand our point of view on this question, but Roy had seen his share of characters, like in the foothills wilderness beyond the rough-hewn mill town of Quesnel. "Man, there were some people out there—*real* hillbillies," he said, shaking his head. "But some of those hillbilly girls . . ."

Despite these fond memories, Roy was distracted by a more immediate concern. "Have you seen my old tomcat around your place?" he asked. "Sometimes he likes to hang around in the sunny field." We admitted that we hadn't, and he seemed worried. The tom, he said, wanders the wilderness looking for a queen, the problem being that there likely isn't another house cat within 20 miles.

"You need to get that cat fixed," said James.

"Sure," Roy rejoined, "but I don't know how to fix a cat."

If Roy couldn't do it, how would it get done? The night before, he had spilled a huge pot of boiling water on his foot. It sounded serious—a trip to the emergency ward for most of us—but Roy simply cooled it in cold water, let it dry, and covered it lightly with a bandage. Similarly, his dog Hombro had wound up with a bear's tooth in his shoulder while defending the camp. Roy had done what he could; Hombro was limping, but the wound was clean and healing nicely.

By the time we were trading Sasquatch stories, Roy's son standing up to measure out with his hands the huge size of the humanlike footprint he had seen in a high mountain valley, we knew it was time to make our way home. Not because we didn't believe—more, in fact, because it was that kind of afternoon, backlit by moonshine and the pleasures of sharing a bottle with strangers who were no longer strangers, that we might believe anything. I thought, for the umpteenth time, of how rarely time and conversation have this generous quality in the city.

"We'll be canning salmon," said Roy. "If you've got some jars, I'll give you some." The salmon, to Roy, were as good as free. The jars were another thing altogether. They meant a trip to town, cash on the counter. The jars were priceless.

Two books ruled the kitchen in Dorreen. First there was my grandmother's increasingly tattered *Good Housekeeping Cook Book,* which was peppered with helpful hints for cooking in the days before electric appliances or refrigerators. Then there was *Plants of Coastal British Columbia,* which began its life with me as a guidebook on wildflower hikes. These days I was drawn more to its detailed descriptions of traditional food plants. Its pages, too, were getting pretty well thumbed.

On the long drive north, we had, of course, made more stops than the one for head-size cabbage and old Willy's tomatoes. We'd camped overnight with one of James's brothers, David, who was traveling south from his home in the Yukon, bringing with him his partner and their new baby boy. I had stored up the pleasure of their company for the long solitude ahead, cooing over Keir as he slept soundly in a sunny patch of grass beside a wild Saskatoon berry bush. We had filled a cereal box with the fat, purple berries, and it was only after two unrefrigerated weeks in Dorreen that they threatened to lose their freshness. That was when I found James outside literally playing paddy-cake, *Plants of Coastal British Columbia* in hand. "Berry cakes," he said, by way of explanation. "An experiment." He had made a mash of the remaining Saskatoon berries, along with wild huckleberries and thimbleberries from the prolific bushes around the house. James patted the mash into two pretty purple-and-red cakes, and laid them on a slab of cedar to dry in the sun. By the end of the day they were already turning leathery.

As August passed, foraged food became an important part of our diet. We spent two hours on our hands and knees in a clearing, gathering dwarf blueberries so dense with flavor that we wondered why they had never been farmed. Berries were almost the whole of our fresh fruit, but still varied enough that we never thought to miss peaches, bananas, or mangoes. The harvest was always astonishing. After noticing a few highbush cranberries on the trail to our cabin, it took little more than an hour to fill three jars. Stored in water, said *Plants of Coastal B.C.,* they would sweeten over time.

It was back to *Good Housekeeping,* on the other hand, to decide what to do with the apples. Decades of ursine pruning had left the three trees shattered and bent—it seemed miraculous that they were still alive, let alone heavy with fruit on every limb. There were far too many to eat; I decided to try preserving some by the "raw pack" method. It was a full-day project, and we chose a rare rainy day to do it. James and I sat peeling apples at the rough but serviceable wooden table, James grumbling as he doubled my output. I shifted my attention to the canning itself, putting a huge pot on the woodstove to boil.

The house soon filled with a smell like apple pie—the jars were leaking. I had no idea what to do, and for once the book couldn't tell me. But in the end, the cooling jars popped satisfyingly to indicate they were sealed. "I think they'll be okay, don't you?" I asked James, and he nodded with assurance, though he had no more insight into the matter than I did.

We had fourteen jars of fresh-picked apples, and it seemed proper to share the wealth. I decided I was willing to stake my burgeoning homesteader reputation on them. "We should take some down to Roy," I said, though I didn't relish another moonshine headache.

"I'll do it," said James with mock bravery.

He came home two hours later with two jars of boiled salmon, and a few new stories that he said he would remember just as soon as he was sober.

I wasn't sure we had adopted the right attitude to our neighborhood bear. As we intensified our late-summer harvest, so did he. These days, when we couldn't actually see him, we could hear him. I wasn't sure what was worse: having our plans for a morning on the riverbank changed by his appearance downstream, or hearing him destroy some grub-filled stump in the forest with the sound of pure, primal power at work. On the other hand, there was the pleasure of watching him from the second-story window, marveling as he shambled through the blackberry patch, nimbly separating the fruit from the thorns with his lips.

We had had our close calls. Once we set off down the path for a walk—our destination, if I recall correctly, was nowhere in particular. We strolled past the cherry orchard where it runs along the river, then through a glade of wild roses and into the thimbleberry patch. Hummingbirds thrummed and American redstarts sang the high notes, and even the old poplar grove seemed to creak with unusual cheer. And then: *Ooof!* A great, deep huff of breath, so low it was like a whispered secret. As one, James and I were backing away, recklessly fast. I couldn't see the bear, exactly. What I saw was a form, a total darkness, like a black hole. The center of the universe.

"Do. Not. Run." James had regained his cool. "Just hurry calmly," he said. We walked backward toward the cabin, then, assuming that no attack was imminent, turned and hustled. We closed the door behind us and put the heavy iron stop in place. We were surprised and pleased to realize that both of us had our bear spray unholstered; James, who had been in front, had even popped off the safety catch.

"Didn't that seem like it was close? Really close?" I asked.

"I think it was pretty close," James said.

We considered the certain rule that people in fear have a tendency to overstate—*that wave I surfed must have been 30 feet high.* We agreed that, at the least, the bear must have been closer than 20 feet. An hour later, when we could hear our furry neighbor in a more distant patch of forest, we went back out to check. The location was unmistakable, a huge depression in the bushes where the bear had been sitting, no doubt munching berries. The hole was five feet from where we'd been standing. I felt sick.

But we were trying to coexist with this fellow creature. He had never behaved in a threatening way—his *ooof* was only an expression of surprise—and I had to admit that he tended to keep his distance, respecting the clearing around the cabin as our turf. We weren't ready to give in to the bearskin-vest approach. The oldest stories of this landscape recommended a different way of thinking. The Gitksan remember fearsome Medeek, the Swamp Grizzly, who punished their ancestors when they became greedy and indifferent to the web of life that surrounded them. They got the message, but then again, they finally killed Medeek with a huge stone ax called a *hegee*.

Thoughts of Medeek and our bear did not offer comfort, but by that afternoon I decided it was safe to bake a pie. I wasn't entirely sure why I had picked this point in my life to become the household baker. There may have been an element of necessity: James considered himself strictly *the cook,* a role distinctly different from *pastry chef,* and this had resulted in a long-standing détente on the matter of dessert. But there was more to it than a pent-up sweet tooth. It was, in a way, a declaration of independence. I was beginning to see that skill in the kitchen didn't have to be synonymous with a housewife slaving over a stove. What would it be like to live in the tradition of the many ladies who had come to Dorreen alone over the years and fended for themselves? I had nothing in particular to escape from in my relationship with James. There was only this: we had been together fourteen years. That was longer than I had done anything in my whole unsettled life. It was the seven-year itch times two.

I was supposed to be making a pie.

The first difficulty in the recipe was "ice-cold water." The Skeena River water qualified, but I doubted anyone would want that much silt in his or her crust. So I jumped on the bicycle to go to the only working well in town. It is the purest water I have ever tasted, and visitors have been known to take jugs home when they leave. James had fitted the old silver bicycle, which we brought in on the train, with brass bells from India to ward off bears. The effect, jingling through the forest, was unexpectedly beautiful and locally famous; that is, Dolsa admired their music. The Buddhist feeling of peacefulness faded quickly as I hand-pumped the water in a cloud of eager mosquitoes. Back at the shack, James had started the woodstove, and I built it up to an inferno—the oven box of the woodstove had to be fiercely hot when the pie first went in.

Everything in Dorreen seems to have this element of guess-work and making-do. Looking around the cabin, it was easy to decide that the place was an accumulation of errors large and small. The worst among these we assigned, perhaps unfairly, to a previous resident named Serge. Serge is known to Dorreen old-timers as the guy who almost burned the town to the ground. One day, they say, he decided he would clear his field with fire. Though this is a popular technique, it is not normally used in the dry season. Frantic Dorreeners rushed to form a bucket brigade from the Skeena and saved the day. We therefore blamed Serge for the woodstove's firetrap chimney that zigged through four 90-degree bends on its way outside, and for the outhouse located just *upstream* of the old well site. We had turned his name into a verb. I dearly hoped that my pie would not be royally *serged*.

A pie, of course, required reverting to our loose ground rules—the flour was left behind from our visit last year. We had brought the butter from Vancouver—it kept surprisingly well with the cool nights—while Smithers had supplied the farmers'-market honey. The apples were from outside the back door. The dough immediately misbehaved, tearing and sticking to the sides of the rolling pin—all those things *Good Housekeeping* assures you will not happen.

"Easy as pie," I muttered. "Maybe it was easy for people who were baking all the time."

"Maybe it was irony," James suggested.

"It sounds like something a man made up," I said.

I repaired the odd rips in the crust, quickly transferred it into the pie tin, then stacked on the apple slices. "Not enough," said James, who had been unable to resist getting involved with the coring and peeling. When I finally, gingerly, draped on the top crust, it could barely cover the mountain of apples. My favorite part was pressing the crust edge with a fork. At that point it already looked like a pie. Then into the woodstove it went, two hours after I had started. This was beyond baking; this was home renovation.

And in the end? A perfectly browned, Fall Fair blue-ribbon pie. I didn't know I had it in me.

On our final day in Dorreen, we walked down to the river for a bath. At least, James planned to bathe; I would wait for Terrace, a motel, a hot shower. Even in the peak of summer, the Skeena flows cold with glacial runoff, and I never get in deeper than my knees. James is surprisingly fastidious about bathing, though some of his other attitudes grow rather more lax over a month in the bush. This morning, for example, he was dressed in gum-boots. Nothing but gumboots.

I was feeling rather wistful as we went out the back door and onto the path that winds down the roots of a centuries-old cedar tree to the beach. The sand is pale beige and ultrafine, picking up even the tracks of birds and voles, not to mention eagles and, this year, a fox that James spotted just once, at a distance. Plovers bobbed along the sparkling water's edge. The air was hot and still, weighty. Then, in the corner of my eye, I saw that darkness. That blackness. There was our bear, a twenty-yard dash away, moving down to the river, a bath on his mind, too, it seemed.

"James," I said, "let's go back."

"This is my last chance to bathe before we leave."

"So what. So you'll stink. You'll also be alive."

James stared stubbornly downriver. He was more than a little exposed, but I could see that he had come to a decision. "I'm going to have my bath. You stand watch with the pepper spray. If he starts to move this way, I can get to the pepper spray and you can get to the cabin."

"This is crazy. I'm going inside."

"Well, I'm going in whether you're here or not."

He was kicking off his boots. The bear, meanwhile, appeared to be going through a similar decision-making process. He stared upstream. Was he going to let these humans deter him? James started to move, slowly, over the smooth stones at the water's edge. The bear moved, too. Then they gave each other a sidelong glance, and proceeded to ignore each other, warily.

Each waded in. James dunked, and the bear plunged under and shook himself, releasing an arc of sparkling spray. James began to soap himself; the bear grabbed a stick as it floated by, and tossed it in his paws as though it were a salmon.

I was still standing on the bank, strangely, thinking how bittersweet it would be to leave Dorreen. When we'd arrived on the train, I had worried about the empty expanse of time that yawned in front of us. Despite all the solitary moments, though, Dorreen made me feel like a part of a larger community, of bears and hummingbirds, butterflies and toads. Bats in the walls. I would miss this ecological whole, no matter how difficult it might be to navigate. What I feared now was the emptiness of the city, the cabin fever of daily routines in an apartment too small for two.

We were going home far richer than we'd come. We had a box of Shenandoah Strawberry apples for cold storage, boxes of crab apples and plums for preserves, two jars of salmon, a dozen jars of apple quarters, three of highbush cranberries. We had two berry cakes and a giant dried lobster mushroom. The Gitksan elders would laugh that we were surprised at this bounty—their ancestors had lived off this land for millennia.

At last James finished his bath. He turned, and I turned, and so did the bear, and we all walked into the forest. Far up the valley, we could hear the train whistle. We had survived the bear, but the spirit of Medeek was preparing to follow us home. These were times of error and upheaval, and the ancient stories predicted the results.

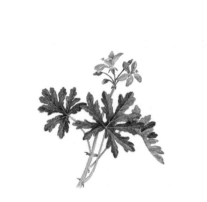

✦ POACHED SALMON WITH ✦ WINE CREAM SAUCE

$2/3$ CUP SEASONAL VEGETABLE STOCK

$1/2$ CUP WHITE WINE

1 CUP CREAM

2 TBSP BUTTERMILK

3 TBSP FRESH DILL, MINCED

2 LBS SALMON STEAKS OR FILLET STEAKS

BLEND VEGETABLE STOCK AND WHITE WINE IN A SAUCEPAN. RE-DUCE AT A MEDIUM BOIL UNTIL ABOUT $1/2$ CUP OF LIQUID REMAINS. REMOVE FROM HEAT. WHIP IN CREAM AND BUTTERMILK. RETURN TO HEAT AND REDUCE TO ABOUT 1 CUP OF SAUCE. STIR IN DILL AND SET ASIDE. PLACE SALMON STEAKS IN A DEEP SKILLET AND COVER WITH COLD WATER. HEAT ON MEDIUM HIGH. ONCE THE SALMON MEAT BEGINS TO TURN OPAQUE, THE STEAKS WILL POACH IN ABOUT 8 MINUTES PER INCH OF THICKNESS. SALMON IS READY WHEN THE FLESH IS OPAQUE THROUGHOUT, COMES EASILY OFF THE BONE, AND FLAKES UNDER THE FORK. DO NOT BOIL THE FISH. REPEAT: SIMMER, BUT DO NOT BOIL.

SEPTEMBER

Just after 7:00 a.m. on August 5, 2005, for reasons that remain under investigation, a Canadian National Railway train jumped the tracks a little more than 55 miles north of Vancouver on a trestle high above the Cheakamus River. Nine rail cars tumbled into the gorge with what must have been a sound like the end of the world. The event could be said to have involved an unusual amount of bad luck. Only three of the train's 144 cars were actually carrying a payload, yet one of those three plummeted into the canyon. It was a tank car filled with 14,000 gallons of concentrated sodium hydroxide solution, better known as caustic soda or lye.

In the world of things officially recorded, the first major development after the wreck was a phone call from the CN Railway to Nexen, Inc., which manufactured the caustic soda in North Vancouver and was shipping it north for use as a bleaching agent in pulp and paper mills. Shortly thereafter, CN began to call the various emergency officials, though, as a later report on "lessons learned" would note, "there were problems with the terminology used in the early messages." A person or persons not yet identified told various agencies the spill was a "leak" that was both "small" and "contained."

It is important to avoid problems with the terminology.

Meanwhile, in the unwritten world, a milky plume was whirling down the whitewater rapids and pools of the Cheakamus. The water, which had been the dun color of brown trout, turned the unnatural misty blue of frozen treats. Tourists at the lookouts along the canyon might easily have mistaken the water for glacial runoff, cool and silty, but to every living thing in the river there was no mistake. Fish leaped out of the water and even onto the banks with their skins burned white and hemorrhaging gills, trying to escape the toxin. Trout, steelhead, char, and spawning salmon were affected, but so, too, were "tough" species like sculpins, lamprey, and stickleback. In places the pulse was so concentrated that it killed instantly; a sculpin was found that had died while attempting to swallow a smaller fish. Later that day, local conservationists dubbed "streamkeepers" would measure pH readings of 14+ in certain parts of the Cheakamus, a reading beyond the scope of their instruments and more alkaline than pure household ammonia or bleach.

The local police received their first reports of dead fish at around 10:30 a.m., or three hours after what came to be called "the toxic event." At 12:52 p.m., an environmental consultant for CN announced that the accident had resulted in the instantaneous release of 10,800 gallons of caustic soda. Half an hour later, the toxic event was officially declared a top-level emergency.

More than 90 percent of all free-swimming fish in the downstream 10 miles of the Cheakamus River were killed, or an estimated 500,000 fish. No records of historical abundance exist for several of the Cheakamus fish species, but the facts were plain enough. For example: there had been lamprey in the river before the spill, and afterward none were observed alive. According to fisheries scientists reporting to a government committee, the spill's effects were "immediate, severe in nature and will be persistent for many generations." No effect on human health was recorded, but this did not prevent one unidentified local resident from telling the gathering media, "Basically, it's murder."

These things happen. In fact, 2005 was memorable for its "environmental disasters," the catchall term that has begun to be used whenever human influence blurs the line of causality for "natural disasters" like the wildfires that year that consumed hundreds of thousands of acres in Texas, Oklahoma, and New Mexico, or the worst hurricane season on record in the Gulf of Mexico. The reduction of a river to a linear dead zone, meanwhile, is rare but far from unheard of. In July 1991 a Southern Pacific train derailed on a difficult stretch of railway known as the Cantara Loop near Mount Shasta in California, spilling 19,000 gallons of the soil fumigant and herbicide metam sodium, coloring a 45-mile stretch of the upper Sacramento River like a rainbow and killing nearly everything in it. In December 1999, massive amounts of a chemical called HMP-2000 were discharged by Guide Corp., an automotive parts manufacturer, into the

White River in Indiana, killing 4.6 million fish over 50 miles. The following year, the Pine River was declared the most endangered river in British Columbia after a crude oil slick from a burst pipeline; the Cheakamus earned the same status in 2006. In a global sense, a "toxic event" like the one on the Cheakamus isn't much of a crisis. Even an hour's drive away, in Vancouver, few people paid attention beyond the first headlines. No one depends—truly depends—on the Cheakamus fishery. The lost generations of salmon can be instantly replaced in the fish shops by salmon raised in fish farms or flown in from Alaska. The Cheakamus salmon will never be missed.

But Alisa and I took it personally. We were counting on a freezer full of salmon for the winter. We had planned to go fishing on the Cheakamus, our best possible option after hearing the bad news about recent history's greatest salmon river, the Fraser. It is necessary to specify "recent history" because, in 2005, the Fraser fishery was once again largely shut down due to a decline in the numbers of salmon returning to spawn, an event for which no one has satisfactorily determined a cause. Most experts agree that a variety of factors have likely played a part. Most, too, would classify the collapse as an "environmental" rather than a "natural" disaster.

It is important to avoid problems with the terminology.

These specific, local losses, small extinctions, and lesser holocausts—we tend to set them aside out of fatigue or, worse, denial. At best we absorb them into a vague sadness over the state of the world. Well, I wasn't in the mood. It was now September, the month of such abundance that it seemed impossible that anyone could ever go hungry, yet my own life felt strangely meager. Alisa had turned so far inward that she seemed hopelessly distant, her physical presence only emphasizing her emotional absence. I was left to guess at probable causes, a labor I knew to be impossible; silence guards its own reasons. All I could do was resist the gravitational pull into darkness. I didn't want the system failure in the Cheakamus to lead my thoughts along the familiar trajectory to a bleaker and emptier world. I wanted to look over my shoulder, toward beauty.

The corner office of Richard Hebda, paleoecologist and senior curator at the Royal British Columbia Museum, is a place of imagination. His desk, when I visited, was pure chaos in a room piled with specimen cases, bottles and pipettes, plant presses, file boxes. There was a bag of rocks on the floor, a wedge cut from an ancient tree weighting a ream of paper. Hebda himself looks athletic, with a fringe of silver hair swept back at the temples. He specializes in tracing strata of ancient pollen back into prehistory, but his office is a gathering point for a wide range of research from across the Pacific Northwest.

"It's true time travel," said Hebda. "That's what I do—that's what I get paid to do." Which is why I was in his office this day, the last before the harvest moon that would rise full and orange at dusk. Hebda is preoccupied with plenitude. There is nowhere better to consider the question. In the same way that the Amazon is a place to contemplate biodiversity, or the Galápagos Islands to wow at evolution, the Pacific Northwest coast is the locus of supersized *life*. Temperate rain forests are home to the planet's greatest biomass, literally the weight of living things. Life here is heavy. The trees alone—the Sitka spruce, Douglas fir, coastal hemlock, and western redcedar—are the largest free-standing life forms of all time.

Humans tend to be a forward-looking species, and so paleoecology—that is, ecological history—is a new science, mere decades old. The first comprehensive history of the North American environment was only published in 2001. The author was an outsider, as is often the case when a new perspective is required; in this case, it was Tim Flannery, a zoologist and visiting chair of Australian Studies at Harvard University. In his *Eternal Frontier: An Ecological History of North America and Its Peoples,* he declares what may be the paleoecologist's first principle: "First we must know what it was like."

Which is a pleasure, in its way. Flannery takes us back 18,000 years, a time span too brief to result in significant evolution of species. The landscape, then, would be in many ways familiar, though organized by a different pattern (sea levels, for example, are more than 300 feet higher now). It is nonetheless a place that modern humans would find otherworldly. For example, the plains were dominated by mammoths, in places living perhaps as densely as elephants in Africa, which can average nearly nine animals per square mile. The mastodon, a smaller trunked and tusked beast but still 15 feet tall at the withers, roamed the forests. Ours was a continent of giants: immense long-horned bison, camels, llamas, wild boar, and three species of ancient horse; huge moose, deer, pronghorn, musk ox, and wolf; and the short-faced bear, the largest meat-eating mammal ever to have lived and a possible inspiration for the ancient Gitksan myth of Medeek. Ground sloths lumbered, and despite a climate not so different from today's, there were lions, sabertooths, scimitar cats, cheetahs, and jaguars in the *northern* forests. Everything seemed to have its larger equivalent, from vampire bats to tortoises. Even the wildest and most profuse corners of our planet today, says Flannery, such as the famous Serengeti safari country of Tanzania, offer only a "framework" for any attempt to envision the abundance.

I was more interested in a nearer history. The age of the giants ended around 13,000 years ago, with competing theories blaming climate change or human hunting as the cause of the mass extinction. By the time explorers from Europe and Asia opened the most recent chapter in North America's story, it was a reduced but still bountiful New World, and its richest corner was the Pacific Northwest.

To begin, Hebda suggested, I might consider how many people lived in the area that is now our 100-mile circle in the years before Columbus put ashore in the Americas. While the exact number is contested, it was certainly high—a study of a single archipelago in one large bay off Vancouver Island found evidence of a past population of 5,000 people. Estimates for the Northwest coast as a whole at that point in history suggest hundreds of thousands, the highest numbers north of the Valley of Mexico. By any measure, the rain coast was no empty wilderness. And all those people were sourcing virtually all of their food locally.

Much of what is known about the indigenous diet comes from middens, like the one that attracted the first settlers to Walker Hook on Salt Spring Island. Some of these ancient dumps of shell and bone are up to 15 feet deep and as long as the Empire State Building is tall. What they contain is equally impressive. The number of animal species the average North American now relies on for food could likely be counted off on fingers and toes; one list of the species found in coastal middens totaled eighty-eight, and included only animals drawn from the sea. Ethnographers did not hesitate to declare the region's first inhabitants "the richest people in North America." So far from desperation were the natives of this place that the anthropologist Wayne Suttles made an early name for himself as the first to argue that Pacific Northwest tribes did in fact occasionally suffer hunger and want. It could occur under certain conditions. One of these would have been the collapse of a local salmon run, like the one that occurred on the Cheakamus River in 2005.

Facts like these might be the best windows into what the world once looked like, but there are still chances, Hebda said, to take actual physical glimpses. I remembered an autumn morning when I was among a lucky few motoring in a rubber raft to the mouth of the Khutze River, lost in the puzzle of British Columbia's fractured coast and one of the least industrialized parts of North America. We entered the bay through a lifting flock of Bonaparte's gulls, some already marked with the black teardrops of their winter plumage. Beyond them, the high tide had buttonholed the river, which flooded its banks and ran deep through the forest. Looking down, I could see salmon swimming through huckleberry bushes and the limbs of trees, salmon drifting through clusters of fairy-ring mushrooms. Dozens of bald eagles watched the surreal spectacle from the bare limbs of a tree. Slipping from the bank, an otter. A herd of seals, heads bobbing, seven of them crowded on a deadhead log. They stared with gathered eyebrows. Had we come to spoil the party?

Had we come to disturb so perfect a world that the seals no longer ate whole fish, but instead took occasional lazy bites out of passing salmon? And the salmon did not end at the water's edge. Their corpses spread deep into the forest. Some of the fish were reduced to drying bones; others were immaculate but for a neat incision at the top of the head where a discerning bear had eaten only the brain. Soon enough we would see the bruins—four black bears, big boars and sows—strolling in sedge meadows the color of lemongrass.

I recalled thinking, *Where have I ever seen anything like this?* The only answers came from the virtual world of Imax documentaries and reruns of *Wild Kingdom,* with Marlin Perkins wearing a too-tight suit on the plains of Africa. Like almost everyone today, I was completely unaccustomed to the kind of earthly abundance that seems scarcely believable in the journals of the early explorers: the buffalo filled the horizons; the passenger pigeons blocked out the sun; the cod were so thick you could walk on the water like Jesus of Newfoundland.

Hebda nodded at my description. Then he leaned across his desk, looking up at me from beneath tufted eyebrows. "The difference is, that would have been *everywhere.*"

I try to imagine.

First, the open ocean. Everything here comes from or returns to the sea. Archibald Menzies came aboard the sloop *Discovery,* an aging naturalist on behalf of His Majesty King George III. On April 7, 1792, he made his first observation regarding this rainforest coast. The ship had sailed, he wrote, into a mass of *Medusa velella,* "a very delicate blue" that stretched from horizon to horizon. It took nearly five days to sail through the sea of jellyfish, while around the ship whales surfaced and blew.

There were whales, yes, and not only the scattering of killer whales that, nearly two centuries later, would be so reviled that an antiaircraft gun was set up near one port town with a thought to killing them faster. Picture the steam vessel *Douglas* in 1868 at the mouth of Baynes Sound, now famous for oysters, as hundreds of humpback whales pass by, their dead-man's songs groaning up through the hull. As many as 600 humpbacks might have lived year-round in the straits and sounds where Seattle and Vancouver are now. They would have hunted the herring. The little fish came in numbers that biologists now call a "mega-stock," but the language of science fails to capture the bounty. Better: fishermen's memories of spawning runs so thick that the ocean floor can't be seen and whole bays turn white with milt. Then there was the phenomenon known as the "herring ball," in which the fish, driven by unseen predators below, exploded at the water's surface with a sound like some massive exhalation, the water boiling silver, the herring caught between the sea and the sky. There is a Haisla story of a time when people were afraid to paddle up a certain passage because a monster appeared to have settled at its entrance. It was huge and white, and when it opened its mouth a maddening cry roared down the channel. The monster turned out to be gulls, tens of thousands of them, feeding on herring. The immense flock would rise and fall on the water, a giant mouth opening and closing.

As the herring spawn ended, the oolichan came, each fish a hand-span long and so rich in oil it could be dried and fitted with a wick through the mouth to burn like a candle. They rushed in vast shoals to the Fraser River, spawning in shallows barely deep enough to cover their backs. These were the images of spring, like the arrival of millions—literal millions—of migrating western sandpipers. Sandpipers in spring, in the autumn, the snow geese, and in winter the endless dark flocks of surf scoters with their bold orange, red, and yellow bills. In their season, the largest gatherings of bald eagles in North America, lining the riverbanks by the thousands. In their season, the black brant geese. The coast pilgrim and artist Jim Spilsbury remembered them "by the thousands and millions," covering acres of the winter sea, or rising as one bird with a sound like thunder to "literally darken the whole western sky."

It is young Jim who stands in an archival photo with, to one side, a huge salmon hooked by his mother, and to the other, the cod that had attempted to swallow the salmon. The two together totaled sixty-five pounds of fish, or enough to serve a restaurant-size portion to more than 120 people. At the mouth of the Fraser River, the place still called Sturgeon Bank, the white sturgeon could weigh as much as a plough horse. Deeper were the rock reefs and the rockfish. Say the names: yelloweye, quillback, silvergrey, rougheye, shortraker, copper, china, canary rockfish. They can live to be over 100 years old, and take twenty years or more to reach puberty.

A drawing from 1902 shows two figures off Pender Island, spearing rockfish from a rowboat. To fish with a spear demands an ocean crowded with fish, nearly bursting with fish, and so does the Salish technique of fishing with a lure pushed to the seafloor with a pole, then freed to toggle to the surface, attracting the *tooshqua,* the big lingcod, to be netted or gaffed. These are techniques for abundance, for the kind of sea that could make a pioneer inspector of fisheries declare, in 1892, "The halibut industry is capable of being increased to an almost unlimited extent," the kind of sea that could annually give up enough halibut to feed 10,000 people a meal every day for a year, and this when the boats still fished under sail. A sea whose immense shoals of spiny dogfish could provide enough oil to illuminate a new century's lighthouses and grease lumberjacks' skid roads into the forest.

The forest. The day before he stepped into it, Robert Brown, a twenty-two-year-old explorer who in 1864 became the first colonial to go by land across Vancouver Island, simply stood on a hill and stared at the dense waves of green fading into the distance. The Europeans entered that dark realm slowly. Even for the Salish the woods were a menagerie of the spirit, with trickster Raven and transformer Bear and the Bigfoot and creatures with jointless legs that chased hapless hunters along the mountainside. It was a struggle just to enter the dim cathedral of green, and Brown's team, when it finally left the natives' worn paths, crawled on all fours or "cooned it" along lunatic catwalks of fallen trees. By night, their camps were haunted: "a wild, weird-like cry"—almost certainly the shriek of a cougar—and the laughter of loons, or a single wolf's howl followed by the chilling chorus of the gathering pack. By day there was meat on the hoof enough that the expedition hunter, One-Armed Tomo, frequently brought back only the hindquarters of the deer. "Eat plenty of venison," Brown would advise future pioneers, "save the flour and bacon for hard time." Grouse and partridge were easier pickings still. "If a man is hungry," wrote Brown, "it is easy enough with a revolver to clean a bush of them, simply by commencing at the bottom and finishing off with the birds in the topmost branches."

But then there were days when the expedition felt cursed, when they saw no game at all. I knew the sensation. I once passed a week in a remote northern park an hour by floatplane from a town that is itself a seven-hour drive from the nearest hospital. It was the wildest place I have known. Yet I never saw more than the distant glimpse of an animal—a bull moose shouldering into a willow stand, a wolf loping down-valley. The abundance was visible only in tracks. Trails, as deep and clear as the finest hiking path, climbed the shoulders of mountains and traversed the plains, hinting at the constant presence of mountain goat, wolverine, caribou, grizzly. Even the muddy floor of a lake's shallow bay was crossed and recrossed by the imprints of moose. Plenitude can be shy. Or not. In 1907 the coal baron James Dunsmuir anchored his steamship *Thistle* on the North Pacific coast and, with a total of four men and a morning ashore, shot a dozen bears, four of them grizzlies.

Those bears would have gathered for the coming of the salmon. Until the salmon have been considered, nothing has been considered. The Pacific coast is a salmon landscape, salmon rivers and salmon forests, and in a "big year," the peak of a four-year cycle, 50 million sockeye may once have moved upstream. I have seen today's great salmon runs. Not only that, I have swum among the fish, their backs breaking the surface around me with a pleasing, constant rhythm, the way you wish shooting stars might appear in a meteor shower but never do. Yet a run of 50 million fish is astronomically greater, a glimpse into an era when a place could be named Catch 'em With Your Hands Creek and settlers complained that the splashing of spawning salmon threatened to swamp their canoes. Every creature that eats flesh would have come to the rivers for the feast. Twenty-two forest mammals are known to eat salmon, more species than most people can name. The fish feed even the soil.

Some years ago I interviewed the first mate of a ferry. He had worked on boats all over the world, but the single greatest moment of natural abundance he had seen had been here in the waters of the Salish Sea. It had been decades ago, and he was on the bridge with his captain, sailing along the border between the United States and Canada, about sunset, and suddenly there were whales; there were killer whales and porpoises; there were herring balls and gulls and sea lions and waves of migrating birds and just so much *life,* such exuberance of life. The captain had idled the engine and they just sat awhile and enjoyed it, letting the schedule go to hell.

Perhaps what he saw came close. Even this, though, is not enough. It is better, maybe, to return to the perspective of the most practical human needs. Looking at the indigenous wealth of the Pacific Northwest, the pioneering anthropologist Philip Drucker of the Bureau of American Ethnology said the following: "Most of the time food was available, and frequently it was so abundant that with the most extravagant feasting they could not use it all up." But then, that is exactly what happened. We used it all up.

Not long ago I had read that even the California condor could once be found on the Northwest coast. Today the last few condors, saved from total extinction by a captive breeding program, cruise the American deserts a thousand miles to the south. I tried to picture the great bird with its bald red head on ten-foot wings, riding thermals over the rain forest. I couldn't see it. I just couldn't.

"Condors, eh? Fascinating. Imagine how much they would have to eat today with all the roadkill."

That even Hebda was unaware that condors were reported in the Fraser Valley into the twentieth century illustrates a key fact about our past. We forget. The effect has been described as a double disappearance. We lose a species, or the abundance of a species, and then forget what it is we have lost.

There are specific exceptions—crows are more abundant than ever, for example, and a person standing on the coast of California is more likely to see a gray whale today than in 1946—but taken as a whole, the living world has progressed in a steady downshift through the generations. The landscape I look on is more degraded than the one my father knew; nature as my father recalls it is a shadow of what his grandfather saw, and so on. The environmental historian Joseph E. Taylor III once wrote that Pacific Northwesterners have been predicting the imminent demise of their salmon runs for 125 years. "One can read these alarms like Alfred E. Neuman and see their authors as so many Chicken

Littles," said Taylor, but he favored the opposite interpretation. "The litany of jeremiads reveals not only the magnitude of the problem but also the fickle character of social memory. Nothing suggests the size of former salmon runs more than the length of time it took them to collapse."

And what is the effect when the average citizen no longer has any idea of what "nature" can look like?

"They have no sense of the possible," says Hebda. "That's an enormous loss. Essentially, we strip Mother Nature to a skeletal form. We still worship and appreciate that, but we don't realize that it's a skeletal form. Not understanding that it's skeletal, we also have no idea how close to perishing it is."

Hebda is an evolutionist, and he considers hope in those terms. Throughout time, life has proceeded through a series of experiments—freak adaptations. Some of these succeed over the generations and others fail, but the flexibility to try new approaches is constant as a driver of evolution. Another essential condition is that the adaptations not progress at the cost of destroying all that is around them, and this is what is genuinely new about our current situation. A dominant freak has emerged, and it is not a life-form, but an idea—the notion that everything can be valued in terms of money rather than the fundamental natural processes that actually keep us alive. The good news is this: it is only an idea.

"We evolved biologically more or less until we got to humans," says Hebda, leaning back in his chair. "We can now evolve *extrasomatically*—outside of the body. We can improve our adaptations, which is what evolution is all about, without having to have generations. The generation time now is the time from one idea to the next."

On a paleoecological time scale, the separation between us human beings and the landscapes that sustain us is brand-new. It has widened in the blink of an eye. For almost all of our history as a species, we depended on our surroundings and abused the environment at our peril. The sudden death of a local river was not a saddening sound bite; it was a life-threatening catastrophe.

The Cheakamus River chemical spill was not going to result in famine for Alisa and me, of course. We had hoped to catch a few fish. But Steve Johansen still planned to take the *Black Heart* out onto the Salish Sea to troll for chum, and we would fill the freezer yet. September was irrepressible. Even the longest-ripening morsels were ready for harvest: hot peppers, sunflowers, eggplants, tomatoes, gooseberries, grapes. Melons. I'd never known that melons grew in my part of the world, but now I knew that September was their high season, and that fact would forever be marked on my mental calendar. I'd never cared much for melon— watery, rubbery cantaloupe. Then I tried them picked ripe, the cotton-candy scent pungent even through the rind, the flesh so sweet that too much of it gave me a headache. Who knew there were so many varieties? Baby sugar watermelon, muskmelon, yellow honeydew, Charentais. I was a melon lover now. A melon fanatic.

But summer ended this month. I turned the calendar and there was October, just its usual four weeks long. By Halloween, the fields would be empty and the world turning the color of rot. Autumn, followed by winter. It was an intimidating notion, the kind of menace that demanded a common front rather than this continental drift that seemed to be dividing Alisa and me.

Hebda, when he gives talks to the public, often suggests something he calls the One Bean Revolution. Everyone, he says, should plant at least a single bean in a windowsill pot. He will always recommend a bean over, say, a tree, because a bean reinforces an original truth: that human beings are sustained by the natural world. The thing we call nature is not, as a tree can be, just something to look at on weekends out of the city. It is what keeps us alive. This is so basic a fact that it seems tedious to say it, and yet this understanding is not among the founding principles of civilization as we know it. There was a time, though, when we felt this knowledge every time we ate.

Hebda, as it turns out, is also a farmer. When he leaves his downtown office tower, he makes his way to the outskirts of the city and a five-acre farm. There the traffic noise is replaced by ravens' wing-sounds and, by night, the hoots of owls. The scientist grows virtually every vegetable I can list. Garlic and dill now come up on his land like weeds. He has grown grain, just to prove that he can, and still sows buckwheat as a winter cover crop. He has just planted his cold-weather carrots—there is no sweeter carrot than one pulled from the ground in January, he says. For the moment, the tomatoes are coming on, and it's been an incredible year for figs.

The garden is a constant reminder that our depleted global environment is linked to the gap we have constructed between our food and ourselves, but a deeper truth is rooted in paleoecology. The science bears witness to changes enormous in scale, the fact that even the continents are works in progress. It can make a person's brief existence seem meaningless; more than that, though, it staggers the mind with the duty of care in our everyday lives. The universe seethed a billion years to give us a row of cabbages, or a quail's egg, or a broken heart. The unfathomable depths of time give Hebda hope. The word has been made trivial, a platitude to deploy whenever there's a need to keep chins up, but "hope" contains a darker seed than that. Hope implies doubt, and the possibility that things really may turn out just as badly as they look.

⇢✳ Poor Man's Capers ✳⇠

⅓ CUP WHITE WINE VINEGAR

1 BAY LAUREL LEAF

1 TALL SPRIG THYME

1 TSP HONEY

¼ CUP NASTURTIUM SEEDPODS

WATER

IN A SMALL SAUCEPAN, BRING VINEGAR, BAY LEAF, THYME, AND HONEY TO A BOIL (WHITE WINE VINEGAR CAN BE MADE AT HOME). WASH NASTURTIUM SEEDPODS AND PLACE IN A SMALL (E.G., 100 ML OR ¼ PINT) JAR. FILL JAR WITH BOILING LIQUID AND HERBS; IF NECESSARY, TOP UP WITH WATER. REFRIGERATE ONE WEEK BEFORE USING. NOTE: USE THE FALL'S EARLIEST, GREEN NASTURTIUM SEEDPODS. WAIT TOO LONG AND THEY TURN HARD AND BITTER.

OCTOBER

It was Saturday night, and cool enough outside that James had made a hearty dinner of pumpkin soup with hints of coriander. The earth could provide that much. And we were finding our way to the bottom of a bottle of Domaine de Chaberton. With every sip I silently toasted my luck that our 100-mile circle was home to some decent wines.

So we were drinking Bacchus, a white varietal originally from Germany, and we were basking. In fact, we were procrastinating. That afternoon we had driven forty minutes to a farm stand for three cases of organic corn—160 ears or so. This chore had used up half of a precious Saturday. The boxes were stacked in the hall, the silks poking between the cardboard flaps. The corn, we had decided, would be our anchor for the winter, just as soon as we got around to preserving it, which we weren't exactly sure how to do. That would be a job for tomorrow.

Because I dimly remembered waving rows of maize in the country garden of my childhood, I was on the phone to my mother.

"We just got an offer on our house," she told me.

My mother's decisions are formed with breathtaking swiftness, and then appear to be utterly unshakable. While James and I had been in Dorreen, she had suddenly left her job as a lawyer—the tenth profession of her life—and, freed from the constraints of place loyalty since her mother died, was immediately on the move.

"How much?" I asked. In a moment that made me wonder if I really had been obsessing over real estate, I learned that I had guessed—to the dollar—the market value of her home.

"Seen anything you want to buy?" I asked.

Well, yes, she had. It was in tiny Lake Cowichan on Vancouver Island, and would cost about as much as she'd get from the sale of her old place in the city. At the brink of retirement, she was passing up the chance to buy low and put away the proverbial "nest egg." She had chosen to trade security for the dream of a water view.

"What are you going to live on?" I wondered aloud.

"Well, that's a good question!" she replied, managing a tone of both apology and defiance. I knew it was no good to give advice, and in any case I was the one who had bought a blow-me-down shack in the wilderness and lived the uncertain lifestyle of the self-employed writer. No pension awaited me, either. The conversation drifted to the real reason for my call: how to put away corn for the winter.

She paused, then asked tentatively, "When did you buy the corn?"

I could sense I was about to look and feel like an idiot. "This afternoon," I said.

"The sugar in corn starts to break down into starch within a few hours of being picked," she said. "It doesn't taste as good, and it loses nutritional value." She was too polite to say the obvious—move it or lose it. She just started describing the process of blanching and freezing niblets. Husk the cobs and wash them. Blanch in boiling water four minutes. Cool in a cold-water bath to prevent a "cobby" taste. Cut kernels from cobs. Pack in freezer bags, leaving a half-inch headspace.

I put down the receiver. My watch read 10:00 p.m. "James," I called out, "we have to freeze the corn tonight." It sounded, at best, like a Mormon's idea of a good-time Saturday night, but he took it remarkably well.

It was fun while we still had a buzz from the wine. Lacking any proper workspace, we set up chairs in the hallway to peel the cobs—to *shuck* them, if we want to be proper. The green husks squeaked as we pulled them back. The corn silk was soft and luxuriant.

I took a break to fill the stainless-steel pot with water, and could barely lift it from sink to stove. Still, I was fond of this monstrous pot, which was proof that the gods of stray things are sometimes listening. For a few weeks in the summer I had thought that we would really need a bigger pot for canning. Then, just as autumn came, I saw this enormous stainless-steel vat beside a neighborhood Dumpster. I waited until no one was walking by—surprised at how embarrassed I was to be a Dumpster diver—and then I grabbed it. It was shiny and pretty much new, and suddenly it was mine.

Bit by bit over the past few months, our kitchen had filled with preserving supplies, whose array and quantity we had never before considered. We now had long wooden spoons and metal tongs inherited from our various grandmothers, along with a magnet for lifting jar lids without touching their edges. We had never found the elusive "jelly bag" for separating juice from fruit pulp, and instead had bought cheesecloth at an ordinary supermarket—we'd assumed it was an archaic product that we'd need to track down at a specialty store, alongside fireplace bellows and butter churns. The slim space between the cupboards and ceiling was now lined with empty jars awaiting our efforts. I'd been elated to find twelve dusty Mason jars for a mere two dollars in a suburban thrift store, each with at least one dead spider at its bottom. I liked to imagine all the successful grandma work they had contained over the years. Later, in a panic, I bought a case of new jars for five times that price. The box was printed with the words BECAUSE YOU CAN, a bad pun that has probably been the company's slogan since my grandmother's cookbook was a new release. Along with the material goods, we'd picked up tidbits of canning etiquette, the first principle of which is, *If given canned goods, always return the jars to their keeper.* Several elderly women had stood before us, heads shaking as they recalled some breach of this sacrament. There were wrongdoers out there, thoughtless grandsons and nieces who'd been stricken from the ranks of those honored with yearly canned wonders.

Soon enough, the lid of the pot was rattling in time to the boiling water, the windows covered with thick condensation scored by rivulets. I began to feel sticky all over, not to mention frustrated to see that it was after 11:00 p.m. and there was still nearly an entire box of corn left to shuck. James's pile of completed cobs was much larger than mine, and I looked at him peevishly. "You're not taking all the silk off." Silently he held up an ear. It was, clearly, as carefully peeled as any of mine.

I said nothing, because I come from a family of silences. We both fell back into the rut, which in its way was a metaphor for everything that might be wrong with our relationship. Here we were, standing around a pot of corn on the cob—a scene of togetherness ready-made for advertising—and yet everything felt weighted with gloomy possibilities.

Fourteen years together. Was I missing out on the last free years of beautiful youth? Had I lost too much individuality? Were James and I too comfortable, too for-granted, too grumpy with each other? What was passion supposed to feel like after fourteen years?

Instead I said, "I feel like part of some apocalyptic cult."

A set of cobs was ready in the pot and I turned to start cutting off niblets with the British carving knife that had served so many roasts at my grandmother's table. Dystopias and privation stories have always struck a chord with me, from the hunted life of Anne Frank to the Cold War threat of nuclear annihilation that dangled over every childhood of the 1980s. "Remember how the Doomsday Clock was set at three minutes to midnight? I obsessed over that."

"I had nightmares," said James.

"At least you didn't have earthquakes to worry about." James had grown up in cattle country, only moving to the coast as he struck out on his own. Since then, I realized, we had lived together within the 100-mile circle we set down on a map for the first time this year. It also happened to be near the shaky intersection of four tectonic plates on what is known as the Pacific Ring of Fire. I was twenty-eight when I finally felt one of the region's frequent lesser quakes. James and I were then living on the third story of a nineteenth-century wood-frame house in Victoria when a magnitude 4.9 hit. I was at my dormer window desk when I felt the whole structure begin to sway on an increasing arc, like a pendulum. James was in the bath and saw the waterline shift. There is nothing more wrong than the feeling of your own house heaving. I wondered, abstractedly, if it was worse to be up so high and fall so far, or to be down below and have everything collapse on you. Yet when the tremors stopped, I was oddly deflated.

Scientists consider this part of the world a locus of instability, underlain by all three possible forms: the unbearable pressure of converging, the dangerous gaps of diverging, and passing friction at "transform faults." The Big One, which is the nickname given to the inevitable earthquake that will rewrite the geography of the Pacific Northwest, is predicted sometime within the next 200 years, which could conceivably include tomorrow. It is both exciting and horrible to know that the earth beneath your feet is constantly shifting.

My whole generation, I think, feels these tensions. No one I know seems able to settle in one calling or one place. It no longer seems believable that there once were people who spent a lifetime working on a single illuminated manuscript. This is an era not of spiritual dedication but of spiritual shopping—of shopping, period. We have delayed or abandoned every form of commitment—from marriage to child-rearing—with the exception of debt. Home renovation is now timed to cycles as rapid as the solstices of high fashion, and we are encouraged to multitask while we drive. There is no *c'est la vie.*

In all of this there is some freedom. We thrill at the promise of radical metamorphosis. I may obsess about megathrust earthquakes, but the End of Oil is a more fashionable doomsday scenario. A whole subculture has developed a certain glee around the fact that, according even to OPEC experts, our global fossil-fuel reserves will last little more than another century at 2003 levels of consumption. Petroleum geophysicists generally agree that oil and gas production either already has peaked, or will have done so by 2010. It is possible that oil will run out in our lifetimes. To look at such facts and see a coming Day of Reckoning, though, requires a leap of faith. A part of us seems to hunger for collapse—for the moment when we are truly forced to change. What we lose along the way—some undiscovered tropical butterfly, or the tradition of returning Mason jars to their keeper—tends to fade with a whimper. The end of the world was too easy. James and I were not believers.

"We agree on too many things," I said, listlessly scooping kernels into overpriced freezer bags.

"We could talk about the sex drives of men versus women," James snapped.

Such are the things that come up when it is 1:00 a.m. on a Saturday night and the wine has worn off and you are still freezing corn.

Food preservation had been less complicated with Deborah.

Looking at the purple-black jars of jam in the cupboard took me back to the late-July swelter of the abandoned railway yard beneath one of the bridges that feed traffic into the urban core. Forgotten places like these are the habitat of the Himalayan blackberry, the laden bushes rising in waves 15 feet high or more. Despite the heat, Deborah and I wore jeans and long-sleeved shirts. I have seen thorns as long as my thumb; I have watched as the vines devoured an abandoned house over a handful of seasons. If, somehow, leaning and stretching for that perfect cluster of berries, you fell into the briar patch, it was possible you couldn't get out. If you were alone, it would be a fairy-tale trap. Held in place by the conflicting snags, bloodied by your struggles, you would have to wait and pray for someone brave to rescue you. But we were cautious, and followed the paths worn everywhere in this happenstance landscape. My fingers were stained purple, and nearly as many berries went into my mouth as into my bucket.

"You have way more than I do," I remarked when my path crossed with Deborah's.

"Picking raspberries was my first job," she said. Deborah had grown up in the Fraser Valley among a tall, blond clan of Mennonites. "I won a berry-picking contest once."

I was clearly out of my league. Deborah, however, had never made jam, so I would be the boss of that part of the job. Not that

I was an expert. I had made jam perhaps three times, enough to discover that the principle was surprisingly easy—boil the hell out of it. When not using pectin, as I never had out of some purist ideal, there was plenty of room for error. It is always impossible to follow the cookbook instructions, which ask you to decide whether the boiling fruit juice runs off the wooden spoon in "sheets" or "drips." While I had never made jam too thin, I had made it so thick you needed to carve it out of the jar. With our 100-mile diet, I had the added challenge of using honey instead of sugar. I had no idea how that would affect the moment of jamming.

"I still hate raspberries," Deborah burst out.

It was a strange thing to say. She had happily agreed to my blackberry plan, and was clearly enjoying herself. Of course, this was not *a job.* The end products weren't numbers on a slip of paper, but jars lined up on a shelf to sweeten the Canadian winter. We could choose when to chat or to rest. We had selected the day to suit ourselves, too: hot but not too hot, with no threat of rain; the trees breathed delicious coolness into the shade. After a couple of hours we decided we were done, and walked home along the tracks, our buckets swinging gently. Farm girls in the city. All along the way we saw others picking berries: women and men of every age and ethnicity, some alone, some with a friend, others with little children. Introduced from Europe, the blackberries have become everyone's favorite weed. This is the only common urban foraging that I know of.

Back at my place we dumped the berries in a big pot and put the burner on low to start cooking out the juice. We added cupfuls of sweetener, following the wisdom of hippie books that suggest using 40 percent as much honey as the white sugar called for. Gradually we brought the mash to a constant bubble, stirred now and again with a wooden spoon. By then, every burner was in action, boiling empty jars to sterilize them. Throughout, we talked of writing, of men, of whether or not we would have children, of places we had visited or hoped to visit. We sipped wine. The hours passed pleasantly, and though I puzzled once again over the thickness of cooling drips on a plate, I picked my moment and called the jam done. The light outside had gone from golden to purple to black, beautiful day to gentle night carried on the sweet scent of blackberries as we poured the hot goo into jars. I hoped Deborah didn't see me absentmindedly wipe a messy rim with my non-sterilized finger. Within only a few minutes we heard the first satisfying pop of a lid sealing onto its jar. Making jam had taken all afternoon and evening, but the last thing I'd call it was work.

It was living.

How have we forgotten this fact? The "primitive" peoples knew it. Anthropological studies of the world's last remaining hunter-gatherers have shown that although they lived in some of the harshest environments on earth, they spent less time working than any typical nine-to-fiver. In his seminal *Stone Age Economics,* Marshall Sahlins revolutionized the Hobbesian view of primitive people's lives—"nasty, brutish, and short"—by pointing to studies that showed the average time they spent collecting and preparing food ran from two hours and nine minutes per day to five hours and nine minutes. "The most obvious, immediate conclusion is that the people do not work hard," wrote Sahlins. Nor did people appear to dislike such work. The Yir-Yiront of Australia, for example, did not distinguish linguistically between work and play. Academics have debated the intricacies of Sahlins's assertions for thirty years now, but his fundamental observation is still respected: "Stone Age" peoples had discovered that leisure could be secured with minimum effort, rather than the series of technological marvels that have never yet liberated us from lives of hard labor. Sahlins called such cultures the original affluent societies.

Today, Americans spend an average of forty-eight minutes shopping each day, and seven on religious and spiritual activities. More than two and a half hours watching television, and eight minutes volunteering for civic groups. A typical commute is twenty-five minutes a day—though Americans suffer through forty-seven hours of traffic jams each year—while 2.8 million people endure "extreme" daily commutes of ninety minutes or more each way. A 2006 search for the longest commute in the United States turned up electrical engineer Dave Givens, who drives seven hours daily, from Mariposa to San Jose, California, and back. A study in the United Kingdom showed that the amount of time people now spend driving to the supermarket, looking for parking, and wandering the lengthy aisles in search of frozen pizzas or pre-mixed salads is nearly equal to that spent preparing food from scratch twenty years ago.

Fast food has come at a cost, and not only in the obvious way that maybe, just maybe, we eat too many Big Macs and not enough broccoli. A Harvard study published in 2003 examined the unprecedented weight gain among American citizens since

ALISA SMITH AND J.B. MACKINNON

the 1980s. The researchers, all of them economists, relied on the broadest possible data—major U.S. government health and nutrition studies involving tens of thousands of people in each decade since the 1960s, combined with the results of the University of Maryland's comprehensive "Americans' Use of Time Project." The clearest explanation for the drift toward epidemic obesity, the study's authors concluded, was "a revolution in the mass preparation of food that is roughly comparable to the mass production revolution in manufactured goods that happened a century ago." Put plainly, we now eat more factory-made, high-calorie snacks. The trend is tightly linked to what the economists call "time cost." Until recent decades, we could rarely consume so many calories in such short order—you could make French fries from scratch, but how often would you actually do so? Before World War II, Americans ate their potatoes boiled, mashed, or baked. These days, deep-fried spuds are America's favorite vegetable.

Since beginning our 100-mile diet, my main snacks had been reduced to, say, berries and yogurt, or celery sticks. Or nothing at all. No more gorging on half a bag of Chunks Ahoy! cookies at one sitting, which I had done in the past from time to time. As the Harvard research shows, I'm not the only one driven by such uncontrollable sugar compulsions.

Despite eating more than ever before, our culture may be the only one in human history to value food so little. From the African scrublands to the Australian deserts, nomads who collected food daily and never stored it considered sharing food to be the ultimate form of wealth. Among the traditional cultures of the abundant Pacific Northwest, a "poor" person was someone who never troubled to catch his own salmon, but was instead content to eat food produced by others. By measures like these, we are nearly all poor.

Of course, thinking about how we use time in our culture is entirely different from actually restructuring your life. We do not live in a world that stops every other activity to bring in the harvest. Putting away food for winter was like adding a part-time job to our full-time lives.

We had put off getting tomatoes until the fall rains had begun in earnest, and the fruits were succumbing to blossom-end rot. It was now or never. We rushed out when a bright gray sky promised that an afternoon in the delta farmlands would be comfortable in only a light sweater. Among the fields, many of them as stubbled now as they had been in spring, we turned at the sign for West Coast Seeds' organic demonstration garden and walked into the shopfront at the head of their barn.

"We were hoping to pick tomatoes," James said to a slightly wild-haired woman behind the counter.

She looked at us doubtfully. "You're welcome to see what you can find," she warned, a little too loudly for the small room.

Armed with a couple of cardboard boxes, we followed her directions into the fields. A farm in late autumn is a somber place, with everything green paling to straw brown and even the sunflowers leaning groundward like palace guards half-asleep on the job. The tomatoes seemed sparse on long rows of plants that had given up any pretense of structure. It was a garden in freefall. Most of the tomatoes were already rotting on the ground.

Our boxes began to fill, however. These fields were a testing

ground for the company's seed catalog, so the variety was for-
midable. Every few yards a marker announced a new type: Early
Girl, Alicante, Big Beef, Black Krim, Oregon Spring, First
Lady II, Kootenai, Taxi, Sweet Million, La Roma. We had no
idea which were for canning and which were not. We picked
them all. Red, of course, but also yellow, orange, green, striped,
some shading nearly to black; elongated or pear-shaped, wee
cherry spheres, monsters with ridges like topographical features.
This final harvest was pleasing, touched by the sense that whatever we picked we were saving from going to waste. Across the
border on days like this, the Small Potatoes Gleaning Project in
Whatcom County sent teams of volunteers into the fields to
gather food for the hungry—over 40 percent of America's
crops, they said, were lost or thrown away. It was another of the
lessons of the 100-mile diet: *There is just so much food.* All the
unpicked berries and potatoes left in the dirt, the "ugly fruit"
that is deemed unworthy of the grocery shelves, the fishheads
that never make it into a stockpot. Since spring we had learned
about all the good eating we had been throwing in the trash, or
at best the compost—carrot tops, squash blossoms, every inch
of the cauliflower plant. Take a single crop: the radish. We had
eaten the baby greens, then the radish root itself, boiled the
later greens for stock, tossed the flowers in salads, enjoyed the
young seedpods as a hot, crunchy snack in early fall. Our in-
ability to feed the world is not an agricultural failure; it is a
failure both of imagination and of kindness.

We lugged our heaping boxes back to the barn, where the
woman eyeballed the produce and then charged us the rock-
bottom price of one dollar per pound. This, too, was a lesson.

Our farmlands are not only our security against hunger, they are also the last redoubt of a gentler capitalism. A dozen is inevitably a baker's dozen, and the numbers on the scale always seem to be rounded down. We've bought fish on the promise to pay later; flowers by karmic donation; honey from an unattended stall. After weighing our tomatoes, the lady minding the store insisted that we throw in a cantaloupe and a few onions for free.

It would have been nice if that heartwarming moment was the end of it. Unfortunately, there were hours more work now that the picking was done. Opening *Good Housekeeping* back home, I learned that we first had to boil the tomatoes for one minute, then bathe them in cool water and peel off the skins. It worked just as described—for half of the tomatoes. The skins of all the others only came off shred by shred; evidently these were not the preferred varieties for canning. Once again the kitchen seemed to shrink, each of us trying to claim some space to dunk tomatoes or wash jars or wield the coring knife. The tomato juice puckered the skin on my fingers. Canning involved a lesson as well: a lot turns into a little. Our robust boxes dwindled into eight quart jars, or enough for perhaps sixteen meals over a winter that might last five months. In sullen silence, we lowered the filled and sealed jars into cauldrons of boiling water where they would cook for forty-five minutes.

I sat at the table with my chin on my hands. The evening had become strained. The whole year had become strained. We'd turned into the irritable couple that is indifferent in private and bickers in public.

"Why do we even bother?" I said.

"Bother with what?" growled James, who can't stand it when what I say is purposefully both vague and heavy with meaning.

Arguments within relationships follow an inverse rule to canning: a little turns into a lot. A squabble about nothing becomes a line in the sand about everything. One comment leads to another and another until the only real question is whether or not someone is going to say, "Bother with *us.*"

A big silence.

"Just tell me," said James as he lifted the lid to see how the tomatoes were doing. He was always trying to do two things at once. "Tell me about your inner workings."

"I don't have inner workings."

"You don't have anything *but* inner workings!"

Did he really want to know? That at any given moment I see everyday life as only *this big,* the space between my finger and thumb. The rest of my mind is occupied with five, a dozen, three dozen other potential lives, each representing some opportunity never taken or currently within reach. Without those worlds of possibility, my life immediately begins to seem boring and drab. I'm thirty-three years old, always broke, and merely *existing* in what, without having been sealed by formal wedding vows, had become a traditional marriage. I had no blues to lament, not really. My only drama was in my daydreams. They reminded me that any day, at any moment, I could change everything, and while many of those alternate lives featured James at my side—the truth was that some of them did not.

I looked out the window. In the unnatural yellow of the parking lot lights, I could see that a dark pulp littered the ground. The trees were growing bare. Autumn on the coast is not the same season as it is in children's picture books, with leaves turning red and gold and blowing down the lane. Here the leaves just fade, drop, and turn to mush. Everything is dying. It is James's favorite time of year—"a serious season," he says—but it brings me down. It is the yearly death of frivolity.

Other things die, too, and when you least expect it. The Fraser Valley had been hit hard by potato blight, and the spuds we had planned to sock away for winter—we estimated fifty pounds between us—had suddenly been lost. When I got the news, I stared blankly into space as the dial tone brayed my defeat. First the salmon, then the potatoes. Now this empty feeling inside. It really was Little House on the freaking Prairie.

> "What good is it to be in town?" Laura asked. "We're just
> as much by ourselves as if there wasn't any town."
> "I hope you don't expect to depend on anybody else,
> Laura." Ma was shocked. "A body can't do that."

The potatoes we'd been able to deal with. I'd remembered the name of a farm in Pemberton, 99 miles to the north in an isolated valley. When I phoned, the good burghers of Helmer's Organic Farm came through with a winter box. Fifty pounds of potatoes wound up in an ugly brown cupboard where James had formerly stored his underwear and trousers.

I was distracted from my brooding by James clattering in the kitchen. He stood over the rattling pot and, wielding the tongs with the air of a sorcerer, lifted the jars through the steam. They emerged, the glass shining, the red globes within glowing as warm as embers.

By some unspoken agreement the night ended there. A box of yellow tomatoes still waited to be chopped and cooked into sauce for freezing, or something like that. *Good Housekeeping* warned that yellow tomatoes did not contain enough acid for safe home canning. Not that we cared about bygone cooking tips tonight. We just wanted to forget and go to sleep, each on his or her side of the bed, with plenty of space in between.

It was almost Thanksgiving. I would be having Thanksgiving alone. James was on the Atlantic coast—another work trip. With a self-pitying sigh, I wondered what I would make.

I couldn't go to Victoria to have the holiday dinner with my family. My grandmother was dead and my mother's world in disarray. She had laid claim to her dream of a waterfront view and was in the middle of moving to her new cottage in Lake Cowichan. I was on my own, and decided to play it safe with a test run a couple of days beforehand. A failed meal on Thanksgiving itself, the harvest feast of our 100-mile year, would be altogether too depressing.

I cautiously approached the box in the hall. The yellow tomatoes had been shunned for more than a week, as though the vegetables were to blame for the current cold war of uneasy gazes and rare caresses in our house. More recently, however, the tomatoes had become a constant, silent reproach. Many would have gone bad by now, but perhaps there was still time to redeem myself with a final juicy taste of summer; all the field tomatoes were long gone from the stores. I opened the box, and a rich smell wafted up, and only a few fruit flies.

Tomato soup was the simplest of things, *Good Housekeeping*

promised, though it involved the tedium of coring and quartering about 10 pounds of tomatoes, minus the third or so that I simply, tragically, had to toss in the garbage. When the chunks had softened over low heat, I cut them again into smaller pieces while they sat in the pot, and added garden rosemary and sprigs of thyme from the plant that had died on the balcony. A little butter, a little of our sinner's salt from Oregon, and I left it to cook until it achieved a soupy thickness.

It was—not bad. Not bad at all. More than anything, it was the leitmotif of local eating: it tasted good because the tomatoes themselves were delicious.

At a loss for what should go on the side, I finally decided on some of our frozen corn and a leftover chunk of butternut squash from the fridge. Again taking my cues from the *Good* ladies, I scooped out the seeds and baked the squash for forty minutes. Finally, I assembled the dinner: the soup in a pristine white bowl surrounded by the corn and the squash on the rim of a plate. It was only then that I realized the entire meal was yellow. I was grateful no one else was around to see.

The next morning I phoned Dave Beers, the editor at *The Tyee,* the local website that had been printing our 100-mile dispatches since June. "I've never seen anything like it," he said, a true compliment from a man who grew up among California's aerospace pioneers in the 1960s. "You're blog celebrities." Various people were trying to get hold of James and me: Could we speak at such-and-such conference? Were we available for an interview? Could we get back to somebody in Montreal, in Norway, in France, with a question about recipes featuring cape gooseberries? There was a growing groundswell of people out there who saw what we were doing as interesting and worthwhile, and likely imagined James and me blowing kisses to each other over organic turkey gravy, rather than me, alone, and him, alone, and the two of us quite possibly on the brink of a breakup somehow loosely connected to the act of canning tomatoes.

I made a joke about my yellow meal.

"You're not going to eat Thanksgiving on your own, are you?" asked Dave, horrified. As a former American he held the holiday doubly sacred, because he practiced it twice: once on the Canadian Thanksgiving in October, then again in November with his parents in the United States. Suddenly I had Thanksgiving plans. "There will be lots of local food," he assured me.

Dave's six-year-old son Quinn was jumping on the leather couch, steadily ignored by his pretty, dark-haired mother Deirdre, who was engrossed in the adult conversation: real estate. Believe it or not, I didn't start it; in fact, I barely said a word. Weighed against the possible collapse of a relationship that was well into its second decade, the housing market and the price of recreational properties seemed paltry. I felt a sudden mental fracture.

I wandered into the kitchen, where Dave was stirring gravy. My contribution to the evening's feast was to be roasted chestnuts. Until earlier in the afternoon, I'd been unaware that chestnuts even grew in this part of the world, but these are the simple, wondrous things that I kept learning this year. I had culled vague internet instructions on how to score each nut with an X to keep them from exploding while they roasted for fifteen minutes. Or maybe thirty minutes; sources did not agree. None of it was actually simple for a kitchen moron like me. The shells were tough and my hands grew sore from gripping the knife for half an hour. I managed not to cut myself. Finally I threw them on a tray and into the oven. When they smelled lovely, I assumed they were done and heaped them into a bowl. According to tradition, as handed down over the World Wide Web, everyone should peel their own; it was supposed to be easy. As I tried one myself, I hurt my fingers pulling at the thick, immobile skin. I hoped no one noticed. The taste: meaty, sweet, tender.

Nora, at ten years old the elder sibling in the family, came over hesitantly and picked one out of the bowl. I was pleased to see the shell fall away easily under her fingers. She nibbled a corner of the nut. Then popped it in her mouth with a smile and grabbed another. "I *love* these," she declared. I was surprised at how I flushed at the child's approval. I ate another myself, and—though chestnuts had never been a part of my life history—felt suffused with communal memory. I thought of the mangled Christmas carol James liked to sing, as his father always had: *Jack Frost roasting on an open fire, chestnuts nipping at your toes . . .* Roasted chestnuts are one of the foods we've collectively nominated to carry a heavy load of meaning, representing time spent with family and friends, one of the few remaining truly seasonal foods. They remind us of times when each season had its special flavors to draw people together, old-fashioned times when talk and silly jokes were everything and enough. Could my restlessness be, rather than a desire for greater motion, a longing to understand how to truly take root in one place?

Soon we gathered in the cheery yellow dining room, the table laden before us. A local turkey was the centerpiece, of course, though it shared the limelight with a tofu imitator for the vegetarian crowd. There was a hush, the uncertainty of atheists before the great meal, the pause where grace used to be. I felt a hollow, suddenly, and my grandmother's absence struck me hard. She should have been at the head of the table, carving knife at her elbow. We should have taken a deep breath, and my sister Robin should lead the singing in her practiced soprano, me following, quieter, my mother quieter still; my youngest sister, Amanda, brasher but never willing to lead; Bryan, struggling to find our high-pitched female key; my grandmother, her gravel voice silent but her contentment emanating outward just as sure.

Be present at our table Lord . . .

Into the silence, Dave asked, "Quinn, what do you give thanks for?" Quinn made a smart-aleck remark, and Dave frowned, though his gaze remained beatific. He turned to Nora, who a little smugly showed up her brother with proper thanks for family and feast. It seemed strange for the first time in my life to be eating Thanksgiving with someone else's family, but it was warm and kind and I was grateful to be in the glow of fellowship, rather than spooning up an unfortunately yellow meal alone.

These creatures bless and grant that we
May feast in paradise with Thee. Amen.

When the turkey and Brussels sprouts and yam casserole had been cleared away, the usual contented lethargy settled in the room. "Nora, will you play us your song?" Dave asked, and she nodded eagerly. Oh dear, I thought, and braced for some enthusiastic pounding on the keys smiled over by deluded parents. "She wrote it herself," said Dave. "It won a prize in a national competition." I was struck by how lovely her simple melody was. *Seaweed.* A song written from her heart and for this place.

I felt a painful nostalgia, as though for a phantom limb. I sat staring at Nora. She was ash blond, thin, pretty I thought. Maybe the kind of girl I might have been if I'd been more self-assured, left a little less free to follow my own whims and drift with the breeze. She seemed, for the moment, like the ideal girl with the ideal life. She would naturally disagree—inside every girl's head is a fiefdom of broken hearts and impossible desires. But it was starting to seem that the way things are and the way you want them to be may in fact be quite close together: within a small circle around your home. A very short pilgrimage indeed.

→✳ SOURDOUGH BREAD ✳←

6 CUPS WHOLE WHEAT FLOUR
2$\frac{1}{4}$ CUPS WATER
$\frac{1}{2}$ CUP SOURDOUGH STARTER
1 TSP SALT

WARM STARTER TO ROOM TEMPERATURE. IN A LARGE BOWL, STIR TOGETHER 4 CUPS FLOUR, WATER, STARTER, AND SALT. KNEAD IN THE REMAINING FLOUR, $\frac{1}{2}$ CUP AT A TIME, UNTIL DOUGH IS SMOOTH AND CONSISTENT. PLACE IN A LIGHTLY GREASED CERAMIC OR GLASS BOWL, AND BRUSH THE DOUGH SURFACE WITH MELTED BUTTER. LET RISE IN A WARM PLACE FOR 12 HOURS. KNEAD AGAIN FOR 5 MINUTES, THEN CUT IN HALF AND PLACE IN TWO BREAD TINS. BRUSH TOPS WITH MELTED BUTTER AND LET RISE FOR 6 HOURS OR UNTIL DOUBLED IN VOLUME. PREHEAT OVEN TO 425°F. BAKE LOAVES 15 MINUTES, THEN REDUCE HEAT TO 350°F AND BAKE ANOTHER 45 MINUTES. INSERT A KNIFE; IF THE BREAD IS DONE, THE BLADE WILL COME OUT CLEAN. NOTE: SOURDOUGH STARTER CAN BE MADE FROM SCRATCH, BUT TRY TO FIND A FRIEND OR RELATIVE WITH EXISTING STARTER; SOME ARE MORE THAN 100 YEARS OLD. FIND OUT HOW TO "FEED" THE STARTER. IF NOT PROPERLY CARED FOR, IT WILL DIE.

NOVEMBER

THERE ARE PEOPLE IN THIS WORLD SO HUNGRY THAT GOD CANNOT
APPEAR TO THEM EXCEPT IN THE FORM OF BREAD.

MAHATMA GANDHI

In the first hours of the month, the morning after Halloween, my mother called. Trick or treat. Her voice had the edge of a person who is close to tears, but feels a need to try to be strong. It had been a long night, she said. Sometime after midnight my brother Sasha had appeared on her doorstep, his face covered with blood, his hair caked with it. He needed a place to stay, he announced, and he'd been in a fight. He had a broken head. A broken hand. A broken life, really.

In my family, this is how people ask if you might want to come home for a visit.

I spent the next nine days in Kamloops, 220 road miles from home and Alisa, who couldn't seem to decide whether she would miss me or not. Kamloops is where I grew up, a place with all the disadvantages of both a small town and a big city. I know: it's easy to come down hard on the place where you endured your adolescence, and to be honest I love the high desert landscape

173

with its tumbleweeds and hoodoos. They are melancholy symbols, though. I do not have fond memories.

I had suspected that the grind of life had begun to overwhelm my brother, and then, with the suddenness of these things, the reality was clear. We were standing in the doorway of the house where he and his longtime girlfriend had tried to hide from their personal demons and where, instead, everything had finally gone to hell. He had given up on her; she had left with their two children. The empty house was now a no-man's-land. These were the blues: even the dog had died. The best that Sasha and I could think to do was take load after load of his former life to the dump.

What kind of year was this turning into, anyway?

For nine days I ate whatever my mother put on the table, the 100-mile diet tossed aside in the face of her chocolate-chip cookies, seven-layer dip, and cinnamon twists. My brother and I drank a lot of that beer I'd been missing, and we laughed a lot while his eyes roamed the horizons, looking for any way forward.

Is it any surprise that I returned to Vancouver feeling like our little local-eating venture was a meaningless distraction? I was tired, stressed out, behind on a half-dozen deadlines, and I didn't particularly care that the first frost had sweetened the kale. Alisa was a sphinx, and if there was any reason that I should whip up something special in the kitchen, I wasn't aware of it. So we had potatoes. Lots and lots of potatoes. Some time ago I had passed through a phase of having trouble imagining a day without them; now I ate them out of dull habit. Of potatoes I had had enough, thank you.

"We need to get some wheat or I'm going to go out of my fucking mind," I said across twin breakfast plates of eggs and hash browns.

"We *have* wheat," Alisa reminded gently; she had stepped carefully around me since my return from Kamloops, where my language had taken a turn for the worse. She was right, of course. We had the tub that contained the ten-to-one blend of wheat berries and mouse shit. Hadn't dipped into that in a while.

Midafternoon, the autumn sun already angling low through the windows, I peeled back the blue plastic lid of the bin and scooped up a cup of the pale brown grains, then poured them onto a cutting board for the ritual separation of wheat from chaff. Clearing a cup of wheat could take more than half an hour, and I sat down with a woe-betide-me sigh. Seeds left, chaff right; seeds left, chaff right. I uncovered a rat turd the size of an olive pit and carried it directly to the garbage. Pulling up again to the cutting board, I was confronted by a curious still-life. At the peak of the pile of wheat berries stood an insect, head lifted to the breeze like a mountain sheep on a backlit skyline ridge. Then he—or she—turned from the summit and began to descend the slope.

"If you want to see a weevil, there's one walking across the cutting board right now," I called to Alisa in her bedroom garret. We had only ever known weevils from novels of the Deep South, in which the insects endlessly invaded the cotton fields of struggling families, with tragic results.

"Does this mean we're infested?" she cried from behind her closed door.

"It's only *one*," I said. "He might have been in there a long time. Come and look. He's kind of cute." It was true: the weevil was small and round, beetling now across the kitchen table, a dark ruddy brow arcing over his snout. He looked both professorial and gossipy, like a television pundit.

"I don't *want* to look," Alisa shouted.

I tossed the weevil out the window into the parking lot, a cruel enough place that I wished him godspeed. Then it was back to seeds left, chaff right; seeds left, chaff right.

Another weevil.

"There's more," I called out, and Alisa appeared at my shoulder. By then I had counted eight or nine. I reached out to touch one, and it folded its legs and tipped over. "Playing dead," I said. Then I saw something else: specks moving across the board, as hard to track with the eye as a satellite across the night sky. Exactly these tiny bugs had been appearing more and more often in the house for weeks—the size of creature that might comfortably set up a colony in your ear. Suddenly we knew where they were coming from. Our infestation came in two sizes, large and small.

"The crop is ruined," Alisa moaned. "It's like *Little House on the Prairie.*"

"It's just a few bugs," I grumbled. "There are worse things in this wheat." Hadn't I read somewhere that old-time sailors used to drop their hardtack on the cook's stove to chase out the weevils before they ate?

Seeds left, chaff right. Alisa muttered her way back to her desk.

But there was a problem. The weevils seemed to be disappearing. I had been certain there were more than a handful. Now I

could see one, two, three, four. Can weevils fly? Another possibility came to mind and I slowly lifted a grain and turned it in
my fingers. Yes. A hole. And nothing visible but the proboscis.

"Oh," I said, this time mainly to myself, but loud enough for
Alisa to hear. "They hide inside the grains."

"I'm not eating it!" she said from her room. "What if the big
ones hide inside the grains, too?" She thought I meant only the
tiny bugs hid in the kernels.

"It *is* a big one," I said.

"I'm not eating it!" she shouted. I could hear that she was out
of her chair and standing at her closed door.

"We have to have something to serve my brother," I shouted,
my sudden anger surprising me. He would arrive in just a few
days, his first visit in almost a decade.

"Sorry about the smell," I said as I led Sasha into the living room
where the hide-a-bed would be his home for the next two
nights. I had, in the end, almost tearfully dumped the tub of
wheat berries into the Dumpster, so many quality complex car-
bohydrates lost in a cloud of dust and weevils. Alisa, meanwhile,
had bleached the walls, ridding the house of most of the minuscule crawlers. The house felt "clean" to us, but now, seeing it
through someone else's eyes, I had to wonder if we might be
starting to seem—*unusual.*

The difference began just a few paces from the front door,
where a jacket closet was now hung with three kinds of drying
chili pepper, along with upside-down bunches of oregano, sage,
dill, and rosemary. I had threaded a line of bay leaves, too,

pinched from a tree in the community garden. Each of these had proved so easy to grow that I now took personal offense at the high price of supermarket herbs; I'd been paying for herbs all my life. Then there was my former clothes cupboard, the one now used for winter stores. The bottom shelf housed a twenty-five-pound bag of organic yellow onions, the first few of which were dusted with mold. The upper shelves held twice that weight in organic russet, red, and French fingerling potatoes, along with some extra Yukon Golds from Westham Island. Most of the spuds had begun to sprout eyes. What these vegetables needed was a root cellar, not a few shelves where I used to pile my underwear, and they needed to be outside in the cold Pacific air, not stuck inside because of a landlord's rules about patio furniture.

There was more. Squash heaped on top of the refrigerator: great carbuncled blue hubbards, smooth-skinned spaghettis, deepwater-green acorns. The kitchen smelled of Dorreen apples—Alisa had thrown a few local Bosc pears in the refrigerator crisper, and the two fruits cause each other to ripen rapidly. By the time I'd rescued the apples, which I'd hoped to munch fresh well into the New Year, most were brown in patches and smelled like hard cider. The rows of canned salmon, tomatoes, Indian plums, pickles, crab apple jelly, strawberries, and homemade "ketchup" were a point of pride, not to mention odorless. But then there was the sauerkraut.

Sauerkraut is the simplest preserve. First you buy a bloody huge cabbage, preferably from a farmer who looks like a German opera singer gone to seed. Next you thin-slice that great head,

toss it with about three tablespoons of salt for every five pounds
of cabbage, and tamp it into a crock, or if, like 99 percent of
modern urbanites, you don't happen to own a traditional ceramic
crock, into a cheap glazed vase from Chinatown. A weighted
plate on top slowly presses the liquid out of the cabbage until it
is submerged in its own juices.

If you're like me, that's when you leave town for over a week,
or about as long as it takes for the cabbage to sour into 'kraut.
Alisa had been left to endure the stench, which is not unlike an
unflushed urinal at the end of a long summer day; and to the
scum and hairy mold, which must be skimmed from the surface
of the liquid every day; and to the fruit flies, clouds of which appeared one day with the immediacy that leaves one in awe of
insect genetics. Cheesecloth was now bound tightly over the
mouth of the Chinese urn with a rubber band.

It was undeniable. The sauerkraut made the apartment smell
as though something had gone bad, which in fact it had. It was,
for the moment, the smell of life, but better anyway than the
smell of dead dog.

I had an image of how the drive out into the Fraser delta with
my brother would be: bucolic, wholesome, earthy, even healing.
Farmers would wave from tractors, and cows would low from the
still-green meadows. Nothing would be as it had been for him.
The air would be crisp and clean, and he would see the world in
its steady cycles, as pleasant as the pages of a children's book.

"That," he said, pointing at a sophisticated greenhouse operation, "is *obviously* a grow-op. And so is that," he added, pointing

to a classic weathered barn that I had to agree was probably blazing with Gro-Lites over budding pot plants. Rural British Columbia is a damaged place, exploited for decades to churn out logs, food, fish, metal ore, and electrical power, then increasingly abandoned as the global economy found places to produce the same for cheaper. The smallest towns ghosted; the survivors hang on to the booms between busts, with a certain percentage of the population expected to live with hopelessness as an institution. And so they take care of themselves. Over the past thirty years, marijuana has arguably become British Columbia's most famous product, a 100-mile herb that organized-crime cops peg as one of the province's leading exports. There are more grow-operation supply stores in Vancouver than there are Burger King outlets.

It didn't help that the delta was wrapped in mist, the landscape revealing itself only in swirls of vapor that made every building seem suspicious or sinister or both. Somewhere above us the autumn sun shone and turned the fog a glaring white. We rolled along Zero Avenue, dead flat against the border. Above us, narcotics officers in helicopters tried to look down through the blankness.

In age, Sasha and I are separated by only thirteen months; my mother cried when she found out that she was pregnant with me, her fourth boy in six years. The two of us grew up fighting: not in a hateful way, but like a couple of bear cubs—it was our nature. We beat each other with fists and feet, and, when our parents weren't around, with books, toys, pieces of wood, whatever we could lay our hands on. Finally we were tossed into judo together, where we learned to bow with genuine respect before attempting to throw each other to the ground and choke each other unconscious. In tournaments, the entire club would gather to watch on those rare occasions that Sasha and I were pitted against each other. We were an odd couple, he chestnut-haired and dark-eyed, with a self-possessed serenity faintly edged by rage and sadness, like a prairie with a storm just visible at the horizon. I, blond, blue-eyed, earnest, quixotic, physically uncomfortable in my own skin. We had led parallel lives almost from birth, rarely treading the same territory. But we observed each other from that distance with interest and care, I think, each of us thinking, *There but for the grace of God go I.*

My little red car bumped down a backroad off a backroad, Sash navigating to a point on the map. It would be a quiet farm, I thought. Chickens would scatter as we turned in, the earth would smell of damp soil, and the air would elicit a peaceful, easy feeling. The place was marked by a rickety wooden sign. Perfect.

Then came a large metal gate and another sign, this one yellow, black, and officious: BIOSECURITY ZONE.

"A grow-op, for sure," said Sash.

Two raging dogs alternated between leaping toward the gate's top rail and spinning circles of frustration on the ground. We stepped out of the car, leaving our doors open behind us, trying to look cool and ready for anything. Sasha is better at this kind of thing than I am.

"Just stop there! Don't come any closer!" A smallish woman had appeared from behind an outbuilding. "One time these dogs tore the gate right down!"

"Is this a farm?" I called out as she approached.

"Yes," she replied cautiously.

"Are you Monica?"

"Oh!" she said suddenly. "You're here for the walnuts!"

Even the dogs seemed to be cooling down, though Monica made no move to open the gate. Once, she told us, a family friend and regular visitor had reached too soon through the fence to work the gate bolt, and one of the dogs had lunged and bit his hand. She asked us to wait and disappeared, returning a few minutes later with two Wal-Mart bags full of nuts. Seventeen pounds of walnuts, a critical protein source for the winter. We got the nuts, and we got the story.

There was a time when Monica was just like me, a person who had never given much thought to where walnuts came from, but who was fairly certain it was not the North Pacific. Her awakening began with a neighbor, she said, who had searched the coast for the best starting stock. After some years he spotted two perfect trees in a backyard in Oregon, a variety known as Manregion brought over from England, which in turn had received its first walnuts from Gallic and Italian traders. The word *walnut* is derived from the Old English *wealhhnutu,* meaning "foreign nut." Monica and her husband still return to those same two trees to get their seed nuts, which take six months to germinate. Ten years later the mature trees finally begin to produce the lime-like fruits that ultimately split, dropping the crenellated nuts to the ground. Because the couple refuses to hurry their nuts with heat, air-drying them takes a further two months. And all the security? That's to prevent anyone from driving onto the farm property who might have an Asian long-horned beetle on board.

"Try a nut," she said.

I pulled one out, passing another to Sasha. Each felt lighter than most walnuts I'd eaten, and I was acutely aware that I held in my hand more than a decade of groundwork. Peering into the fog, I could see only one tree, a latticework of smooth gray limbs hung with big oval leaves turning black on the boughs.

"I don't have a nutcracker," I said. Monica smiled, and I saw now that she was younger than I'd thought at first, blue-eyed and with straw-blond hair jutting out from beneath a toque. She stepped through the gate, causing Sash and me to tense as the dogs tried to press past her knees. Reaching into a bag, she pulled out a nut. Pinched it between forefinger and thumb. It popped open.

I tried her trick, and sure enough, these Manregion nuts were thin-shelled, snapping open with a squeeze. The inner architecture of the nut was also simpler than in familiar store-bought nuts. It was easy to pull the whole nut from the half-shell. "They're a bit sweeter than the walnuts you'll know. Less bitter," she said as we took them in our teeth. The first taste was a pure freshness, a perfect moistness, and finally a sweetness. The texture was meaty but leaning just far enough toward crunch, and only in the aftertaste was there a hint of that familiar walnut bitterness, in this case just enough to leave the mouth feeling clean.

"I think this is the best walnut I've ever eaten," I heard myself saying.

I looked over at Sash, and his face was a mixture of enjoyment and reluctance, as though he wasn't ready, not yet, for simple pleasures. He was anchored in his ordeal, but was it possible, might it even be fair to say, that this perfect walnut, this November mist, the cold disk of sun in the sky, was a first glimpse of a fairer shore? It might be saying too much. Sometimes a walnut is only a walnut.

"I think it is," he allowed carefully. "I think it is."

We paid, and said our good-byes. The drive home took us past a favorite vineyard, Domaine de Chaberton, where we stopped for a leavening sample or two of Bacchus, chardonnay, and Madeleine sylvaner, the grapes themselves growing nearby somewhere in the murk. We walked out with a mixed case of bottles. Good wine, too, is useful for seeing the world with new eyes.

At home, I carried the walnuts; Sasha lugged the wine. We bumped through the front door, smelled the sauerkraut, saw Alisa in a steamy kitchen putting something into jars.

"How was the walnut farm?" she said, something irrepressible in her smile.

"Foggy."

"I have some news you're not going to believe," she said.

"You're pregnant," said Sash.

"Much, much better."

I couldn't think of the last time I had seen her eyes dancing like this. A long time. Too long.

"I found a wheat farmer."

I only know wheat in one image: sprawling, god's-country fields that stretch horizon to horizon underneath a golden sky. Highland House Farm looked all wrong. Seen from the road, it might have been a polo club poised on the English downs. Our wheels crunched on a long driveway lined with hedges that gave way here and there to a pasture furred with green. Coming up a dirt track was a tall figure accompanied by a black Labrador puppy collared with a red kerchief.

"Welcome to the farm," said Hamish Crawford in the softened Scottish brogue of a longtime émigré. Hamish had been quick to invite Alisa and me to the farm when we'd called, though we had failed to give fair warning of our hope, fairly desperate at this point, that he would have some flour for us. As potential saviors go, he inspired confidence: gum boots, a hood poking out from a blue plaid macintosh, a silver buzz cut and muttonchop sideburns that linked into a brush mustache. He looked toward his grazing sheep with fondness and called them "woollies." A real farmer.

"Most years we've found four acres does it," he said. "With four acres planted we'll get 32,000 loaves' worth of production."

Alisa and I gaped at each other. This small field? Thirty-two thousand loaves? Suppose an average household puts back two loaves of bread a week. This field—this field alone—could supply 300 homes with bread for a year.

Hamish's flour goes into a bakery, The Roost, on the corner of his land, which is managed by another family and employs a handful of staff. It is a perfect, closed-circle economy. "If I can get *that* full," he said, pointing to a galvanized silo perhaps thirty feet high, "or even two-thirds full, we're good for the year."

I had expected Hamish's operation to be the eccentric project of an obsessive who works with arcane varieties of eighteenth-century wheat and prepares his compost in the skulls of goats. But Hamish holds a degree in agriculture from the University of Edinburgh in Scotland, and has experience wheat-farming in the Canadian breadbasket. He grows hard red spring, one of the dominant commercial varieties in North America, and "just throws the seeds into the ground." Because of the microclimate of the Saanich Peninsula on Vancouver Island where he farms, his land is drier in the summer than many locations on the Great Plains. "I actually find growing wheat is *easier* here than many places," he told us. "I know that's a huge surprise to most people."

A thin, cold drizzle began as he led us into the outbuilding that houses his fanning, hammer, stone, and sifter mills, along with a tractor whose engine parts were laid out in grease on a cement floor. He laid his hands on a plastic bin, tugged at the lid—and there it was. One-hundred-mile flour. The color of linen. "That's the stuff," he said, almost to himself, then took a scoop in one rough hand. He offered us each a pinch, then studied our faces as we realized this was not the flinty, almost flavorless powder we'd always known, but something layered and complex, a taste that promised to fill a house with the odor of fresh-baked bread. Hamish took a dab himself, then cupped his hand to his puppy, which licked away the rest.

"North Americans are bad," he said. "They damn near forgot how exciting eating can be." At Highland House, he said, he can get apples, veggies, wheat, berries, sheep's wool, mutton, chicken, even ostrich meat and the giant eggs that can serve a dozen people. "There is always something on the dinner table that comes from the farm or a friend. You can sit down to every meal and be excited about it. You don't ever have to sit down for a meal and just go *blah.*"

Hamish was sealing the flour tub again, turning to step back into the rain. The visit was coming to an end. I spoke up.

"One thing we're wondering is, well, we've been trying to eat only within one hundred miles for a year, as you know, and you're the first person we've met who farms wheat . . . is there any way we could buy a bag from you—"

"We'll pay you," Alisa cut in, "anything you want."

"Of course I can give you some flour," said Hamish.

"That's great." Alisa and I spoke at the very same time.

"I can't give you any right now, unfortunately."

We both blinked.

"I have those engine parts out, and if I grind the wheat, they'll be covered in flour. Call in a week or two. Give me a few days' notice and I'll get you some."

We could hardly be disappointed. We had waited seven months for flour; we could wait a few weeks more. Besides, there was a consolation prize: two loaves of dense, chewy, stick-to-your-ribs sourdough from The Roost that somehow tasted exactly like the dew and sea breezes of a particular sleepy hollow in the middle of the Saanich Peninsula.

We enlisted our friend Adrienne, a regular visitor who lives on Vancouver Island, as the most likely carrier for our eventual wheat. Adrienne is one of those people who seems to live enough for a dozen of the rest of us, and when she's not rock climbing she is twirling flaming torches, and when she's not twirling flaming torches she is onstage in an amateur theatrical production. She does all of this while awaiting her date for the full knee replacement she needs from her arthritis. She entered into our local-flour scheme with enthusiasm on the promise of a plate of 100-mile pancakes.

Meanwhile, there was plenty to do. The overripe Dorreen apples hit a crisis point, and we passed most of a Sunday afternoon coring, slicing, and canning them as applesauce. Mornings were a delight of fresh—can you say "fresh" about something that's gone bad?—sauerkraut fried with eggs and potatoes. I made phone calls home, where my brother was fighting for his children with a first hint of the return of his old calm strength. I spread walnut pesto over fried zucchini. One afternoon I talked to a woman in northern British Columbia who, with her teenage single parents' program, had put together a thirteen-item 100-mile lunch centered around elk burgers, and who, when she found out we were still eating meals of potatoes, potatoes, and more potatoes, had this to say: "There're all these stories that used to come out of Ireland about, you know, five people sitting around a table eating maybe five potatoes. The idea was to chew the potatoes very slowly and imagine they were something else." It is a comfort to have allies.

Then came the message from Adrienne: she was coming across to Vancouver to visit her grandmother. I reached for the phone.

A few days later, we got the word:

Subject: Flour

The flour is ground and ready to go for this weekend. It can be picked up at the bakery anytime.

Enjoy!
Hamish

I patched the news through to Adrienne, feeling like a nineteenth-century telegraph operator:

Subject: Flour!

I've just heard from Hamish Crawford about the possibility of flour . . . it's a go! Send in the team!

She let us know that she would make it to Highland House that weekend, weather willing. November had turned unusually cold. Within twenty-four hours, radio forecasters were announcing a massive snowstorm building on the Pacific. I sat at my computer, compulsively checking satellite images that showed a dense wall of weather inching toward Vancouver Island.

"We could rent her a four-by-four," I said seriously, as the mare's-tail clouds that foretell a tempest feathered their way over Vancouver. Today was the day.

"Sure," said Alisa. "A Hummer to pick up our hundred-mile wheat."

By noon the freezing rain was dumping down on Vancouver in huge, wet lumps, and the city was loud with the boom of fender-benders and the wail of sirens. We tried calling Adrienne, worried that she would risk life and limb to get to the farm. She wasn't home. Maybe we shouldn't have been so dramatic, we thought. It was only flour, for god's sake. It might have founded Western civilization, but it was only flour.

We went to bed in a city silent with snow.

And woke up to this message:

Subject: The Eagle Has Landed!

We were the proud owners of 75 pounds of flour, enough for 150 loaves of bread or more pancakes than anyone could count. We also had new furniture for the house: three tall, sealed pails. On one, containing an unsifted grind with all its bran and germ intact, Hamish had written three words.

"The Real Thing."

There was more that needed to be done, I suppose. Winter was suddenly here, and we should have canned some sauerkraut or, I don't know, smoked some salmon or started making yogurt. Instead we heated the apartment with baking: bread, biscuits, pies, pizza dough, tortillas, even crackers. I had never given any thought to where crackers come from, and had to admit I was surprised that they were *baked*. We were back in the familiar world of carbohydrate loading, and yet it was not the same. I had never imagined the difference fresh flour would make. Everything we made we ate simply, letting the flavor of the wheat stand alone. It tasted—*ancient*. We would sit together to break the bread. A sacred act.

And one night, the house full of good smells, the snow outside refusing to melt away, the calendar ready to turn to December and a long winter, the phone rang.

"Hello?"

"Hey."

It was Sasha. For the first time in years he sounded just like the brother I used to love to fight.

⇥⊁ Maple Walnut Crêpes ⊁⇤

1 CUP SIFTED FLOUR

$\frac{3}{4}$ CUP WATER

$\frac{3}{4}$ CUP MILK

3 EGGS

2 TBSP MELTED BUTTER

$\frac{1}{4}$ TSP SALT

2 CUPS WALNUTS, SHELLED AND CRUSHED

BIGLEAF MAPLE SYRUP

WARM A PLATE IN THE OVEN AT 150°F. IN A LARGE GLASS BOWL, WHISK THE FIRST 6 INGREDIENTS INTO A WELL-MIXED BATTER. LIGHTLY GREASE A LARGE FRYING PAN WITH BUTTER. HEAT UNTIL A DROP OF WATER BOUNCES ON CONTACT. LADLE BATTER INTO THE CENTER OF THE PAN, TURNING THE PAN OR USING A SPOON TO SPREAD THE BATTER INTO A THIN, LARGE ROUND. WHEN THE BATTER HAS COOKED THROUGH AND BEGUN TO STEAM, CAREFULLY FLIP THE CRÊPE. FRY A FEW MOMENTS MORE, THEN SET ASIDE ON THE PLATE IN THE OVEN. REPEAT UNTIL THE BATTER IS USED UP, KEEPING THE GROWING PILE OF CRÊPES COVERED WITH A CLOTH. TO PREPARE FILLING, STIR SYRUP INTO WALNUTS UNTIL COATED. ROLL $\frac{1}{4}$ CUP WALNUT FILLING IN EACH CRÊPE. SERVE WITH BUTTER AND SYRUP ON THE TABLE.

DECEMBER

"We were canoeing to that island, where there's a freshwater spring bubbling up." August Sylvester, sixty years old, was pointing south into the maze of the Gulf Islands. As a boy he spent much of his time on the sea with his grandfather, gathering food and visiting far-flung family. Now he was standing on the beach where he was born, on Kuper Island, which is an Indian reserve of the Penelakut tribe of Coast Salish. Sylvester is not a large man, but heavyset and strong looking. He used to make his living as a carpenter, and now carves wooden traditional figures such as salmon and hummingbirds to sell at summer markets. His wide face is topped by a blue baseball cap embroidered with a tribal hoop and feathers. "My grandfather was filling up our water jugs, and talking Indian," continued Sylvester, adding a few sentences in his Hul'qumi'num language; his words in English retained its lilting inflections. "My grandfather told me, 'Someday you'll have to *buy* water.'" Sylvester shook his head at the memory. "In the days coming, only rich people will be able to afford to eat."

We were standing on a long, sandy spit licked by the Pacific. Sometimes I think this landscape is most beautiful in the winter: blue-gray mist, black forest, steely ocean, a horizon overlaid with islands large and small, receding like longing and memory. Kuper itself is a small hump of land rising from a channel and swathed in dense coastal firs. A well-worn village overlooks the ferry that crosses to and from the looming mass of Vancouver Island. Over the past decade, other Gulf Islands have become retreats for Microsoft millionaires and rock-and-roll executives. On Kuper Island, the median annual income is $8,112. But in some ways, Sylvester said, living on an island apart was a blessing. "We teach our children the Indian language, Indian ways. Our culture is strong," he said to me soon after I drove up a potholed dirt road to his double-wide trailer home. The village of 300 people seemed to have no street signs or house numbers, and I'd only found Sylvester's home when a friendly stranger in a minivan offered to lead me there.

I was on Kuper Island by chance—an unexpected assignment to write about the Gulf Islands. It was my turn to wander while James lingered alone at home, disappearing into his work and never at a loss to take care of himself. I had never been to Kuper, and while I was eager to pick out the details that make each of the many islands unique, I knew, too, that whatever I learned would somehow come back to food. More than other places, islands have always had to fend for themselves.

The beach beneath our feet was made from thousands of years of discarded shells—we were standing on the hangover from millennia of feasting. Sylvester pointed toward the channel. His grandfather had only a small boat, he said, and he remembers how the old man would speak to the humpback whales as they passed. None have come by for decades. Back then, this beach had been the place to go for black mussels, "a real delicacy." They're gone now. The same with the red sea cucumbers, which used to be his favorite breakfast food. "We'd roast them and they were real sweet. Just like they'd been sugared," he said. Now, breakfast is cereal. Everything that disappeared was replaced with something from the supermarket.

I tried to imagine a child savoring a sea cucumber. I had seen green ones once as a young teen on a field trip to a biological research station; they were droopy, foot-long sacs that I squeamishly cut lengthwise with a razor at my teacher's instruction. That it might be roasted and eaten never entered my mind. Then again, at that point in my life I'd never gutted a fish or even touched raw chicken. Such is the life of the modern teenager.

Sylvester could point to nearly every place within sight, north and south, and tell what used to be harvested there. That was where they caught the spring salmon in December, he said, gesturing, and there they netted the pencilfish in May; in the channel toward Chemainus, there were always shrimp and prawns. This spit was evidently once the center of village life.

"People got to buy stuff now that was free. We used to trade for food, we never bought it. We've got an easier life now, with electricity and freezers. We don't need to go after food every day. But we're weaker Indians because of it. Now people think you have to be pretty poor to pick food off the ground as we did.

"I learned to hunt when I was six years old. We're in a different time, a lazy time. We don't go fishing or hunting no more. We don't row no more." The old canoes were thirty feet long, he said, and held as many as a dozen people. Then, Kuper was a launching point to new vistas and adventures. Today the island has closed in on itself, to its three and a half square miles and two small villages. People wait for the ferry, or for the money to pay for the ferry. "Now we've got fast cars and telephones. We don't visit anymore. I speak my language—but who am I going to speak it to? We're going to lose our history and way of life."

"Aren't people interested in the old ways?" I asked.

"Outsiders are, like you," he said. "But the kids would rather watch TV."

He stared east across the water, then noticed, with evident surprise, that there appeared to be houses on what he thought was a part of the Penelakuts' reserve land. It was clear that he hadn't been to this beach, the beach where he was born, in a long time. His attention shifted to a small pincushion island bristling with trees. "That was where we put our dead," he said with dark satisfaction. "No one's built a house *there* yet."

A light rain began to fall. To another coastal native group, the Haida, a beach like this one was their original place, pure and blameless, where the first humans climbed out of a clamshell. A moody, temperate Garden of Eden. I had always found these smooth midden beaches pretty—some are so white they hurt your eyes in the summer sun—but finally they said something to me. This place, my home, this coast of green and rain—this was where I had climbed out of a shell and begun to exist.

"Well, I guess that's it," Sylvester said abruptly, and we trudged back to my rented car, our feet sinking in the sand.

I was holding a TV dinner, awash with mixed feelings. Guilt, of course, though I was still on the road, away from James, and had our 100-mile diet travel clause to fall back on. At the same time, I admitted to myself that I was looking forward to the promise of convenience. Open the box, put it in the microwave, it's ready to eat. We're in a different time, Sylvester had said, a lazy time. In fact, I didn't even have to do so much. I was visiting my grandmother Dena, and she wanted to serve me dinner, and this was her way of doing it. She didn't cook much anymore.

I haven't lived near my father's mother since shortly after he died twenty years ago, when Dena still made delicious ox-bone soups and apple pies for Sunday dinners in the prairie city of my childhood. She still lived in Edmonton, where nearly a million people dwell at a latitude farther north than Ulaanbaatar, Mongolia. My grandfather had died two years back, and Dena had moved into a senior's apartment. From the window beside the elevator I could see Pleasantview cemetery, where my grandfather was buried. Their old house was just beyond it, a fifteen-minute walk away. Every instinct Dena had was to keep everything precious and familiar close to her. There seemed to be only one exception. Without Walter, she seemed to have lost interest in cooking.

I handed my grandmother the box of frozen shrimp penne and drifted back to my chair in front of the television, where *Everybody Loves Raymond* flickered on the screen. It was unseasonably warm tonight for Edmonton in December, but still cold enough for frostbite with the chill of the prairie wind. I could hear her opening the box, and the square clunk of the microwave door.

Strangely, I felt linked to the TV dinner by family history. My grandfather Walter's kin played an unintended role in the development of the global food trade. They hailed from the Scottish village of Crail, on the Firth of Forth, which reaches into Edinburgh. Walter's mother, Hannah, was an itinerant midwife, and his father, William, a fisherman with a rough-and-tumble past. There were only two kinds of men in Scotland's villages at that time. The first never left home—an old story from the county tells of a man who, when asked if he'd ever been abroad, replied, "Nae, but I ance kent a man who had been to Crail." William was the second sort. At the age of twelve, lacking money and stepmotherly love, he ran away as a sailor on the English tall ship *Thermopylae.* By the time he was sixteen, he'd seen every major port in the world. The men of the *Thermopylae* filled and emptied her hold of every resource the British Empire could acquire: wheat from America, wool from Australia, timber from Canada, rice from Japan. Above all, tea from China.

Tea was the fast clippers' raison d'être, as the quality of the valuable leaves deteriorated over time. The *Thermopylae* garnered world records for speed—China to London, ninety-one days—as it rushed the national beverage home.

The mark of an empire, it seems, is to eat its length and breadth. In Roman times, food grown within the Italian heartland was considered suitable only for peasants. For a feast meant to impress, a guest might find laid out in one sitting peacocks from Samos, grouse from Phrygia, cranes from Ionia, tunnyfish

from Chalcedon, eels from Gades, oysters from Tarentum, sturgeon from Rhodes, wheat from Africa, and spices from India and
China. However, it was the British mania for the perfect cup of
tea that built a global trade of the greatest speed the world had
ever known.

The first refrigerated ships that allowed perishables such as
meat and cheese to move transcontinentally appeared in the late
1800s, and they were steam-driven rather than sail-powered.
Many of the sailing men scorned the innovation. Steamship men
were never heard to sing a shanty, they said, because there was
nothing joyful about such work; and if men fell asleep on the job
and caused disaster, well, who could blame them? I will never
know if my great-grandfather William said these things, but his
actions suggest that he might have. When the days of sail ended,
he stayed home and built wooden yachts for a wealthy patron
after whom both my grandfather and father were named. The
outmoded *Thermopylae* was decommissioned in his lifetime—
sunk offshore of Portugal in a blaze called a "Viking funeral"
in 1907.

Food had traveled farther and farther from my grandmother
for most of her life. Her girlhood in a coal-mining town near
Newcastle was as opposite as could be from that of my grandmother Margaret, who had died just months earlier. Margaret
was raised with a maid at hand; young Dena's fondest dream was
to *be* a maid. It sounded like a pleasant life, she thought, sleep-
ing in a mansion with all your food and clothes supplied. Her
mother was enraged when she learned of it. "You will never be a
servant," she said through clenched jaws; she herself had been
raised in a London orphanage, and had gone into service as a

teen. She had later married a coal miner, vowing to live an independent life even if it must be poor.

Dena was a child through the national strikes of the 1920s when food was scarce, and a teen in the Depression when food was even scarcer. Then came the rationing of the war years—belt-tightening was all she ever knew. Still, she recalled the pleasures of eating from home ground. Her father's garden brought him contentment during the daylight hours he was free from the mine: the family enjoyed the annual progression of onions, turnips, carrots, leeks, and celery. Picking raspberries, blackberries, currants, gooseberries. Chasing a boiled egg down a hill at Easter. Buying cockles from itinerant vendors in summer. She still remembers the name of her favorite strawberry variety—Climbing Kruger Climax, a saucy name and "sweet as honey." When she told me this, I realized it was the first time I had ever heard a strawberry called by its varietal name.

She, too, saw her world widen through food. It gave her her first job, and the means to her first real taste of "away." As a teen she worked in what she describes as a "high-class fruit stall," where she brushed the sawdust from grapes as she unpacked them from barrels, and carefully arranged banana bunches for display. She rode her bicycle 40 miles a day for the privilege of twelve- to fourteen-hour shifts, six days a week. She became as fit as any modern-day racer. On Sundays her cycling club explored the countryside: 75 miles, 100 miles, 150 miles. It was the farthest she had been from her home in her life. Still, she couldn't imagine that a time was coming when the beloved English apples she still recalls—Jonathans, Gravensteins, sweet-fleshed Russells from the south, Bramley Seedlings for cooking, and so many more—would vanish from the grocery stores, even at the height of apple season. There was so much demand. Her shop stayed open late on Saturday nights because people liked to buy fruit as a treat when they went to the movies.

Though these humble luxuries were available to most people, no one she knew owned a car, and families did their laundry in sheds out back, where they heated a tub of water on a fire. "It was like medieval times, the way I grew up," she told me, smiling wistfully and shaking her head. "We lived like people had always lived."

Ping! The microwave announced that our penne dinners were ready. My grandmother ceremoniously placed the plastic trays on the brown-and-gold folding TV tables that I remembered from my childhood visits to her house. I dug into the glistening pasta and believed, briefly, that the food was good. But I felt unnourished. I was spoiled from eight months of good food, fresh-picked or home-canned. I craved 100-mile meals, no matter how many potatoes they might involve. That food made me feel alive.

My grandmother settled into her brown La-Z-Boy recliner. She stared dispiritedly at the screen as an old *Seinfeld* came on, but decided to watch it anyway. At the commercial break she pressed the mute button. "Will you take me to Wal-Mart tomorrow?" she asked. "I would like to get a new lamp."

I am already old enough to ask myself how times have changed so much, so fast. The drive to the Wal-Mart would inevitably take us past endless big-box strips. I could remember when all of it was farms and weathering grain elevators. Was I, too, at the tail end of generations that had forgotten their "old ways"?

Certainly, I was affected before I was even old enough to understand. Way back when I was four, I became increasingly sickly and spiritless. My mother took me to the doctor, who poked and prodded and deliberated. In the end, he pronounced, "She's depressed." Depressed, at four years old. Why? No one had an answer. Later, as a teen, I was struck by Susanna Kaysen's memoir *Girl, Interrupted,* in which she describes the treatment of her depression through electroshock therapy. Afterward, her thoughts glided pleasantly like a figure skater through her mind, always evading the center where the darkness lay. I thought that sounded lovely. I have long evaded the real reasons for my discontentment. I still can't tell what they are, precisely, but I feel their presence most acutely in moments like this one with my grandmother, imagining a day in a big-box store that had replaced an old farm.

By contrast I could see more clearly the times when, over the past months, I had been genuinely happy. Picking strawberries, eating the first salad from our tiny garden, riding my bike to the farmers' market, admiring the miracle of risen dough. The moments were so simple I'd hardly noticed them at the time. I realized, too, that James was a part of all those memories. So often when I was with James, I was laughing. Like the countless times I sat at the table to keep him company as he cooked, and he did the jerky jig he calls his "kitchen dance." It was wonderfully ridiculous.

"Sure," I said to my grandma. "We'll go to Wal-Mart."

—

"Notice that smell?"

James was peeping with mock fear from under the covers beside me. After the Gulf Islands, and my grandma's place, and finally my mother's new waterfront cottage, I was home. Our humble flat seemed somehow larger than I remembered. I liked its big windows and hardwood floors and the bamboo stalks that screened the barn-red Edwardian home across the way. I liked the whispering snow that made the two of us nestle beneath the blankets.

"What smell?" I said.

"Like tangy ranch dressing."

I poked my nose out into the cold morning. "What do you think it is?"

"The onions going bad," he said.

All I could do was sigh. At least three more months of winter to go. In the future, every apartment block will have a huge root cellar, the way each has underground parking today. Without that archaic luxury, I would have to put the 25 pounds of onions in an old pillowcase and hide them away in the black plastic bin we kept on the balcony in defiance of landlord rules. Maybe the cool air would arrest their decline, or maybe all the moisture would make them rot faster. Lacking wisdom, I prayed for luck.

The weather was not cooperating with our 100-mile year. Snow is rare here, but when it comes, it's as prodigious as the rain. The novelty breeds panic—cars skitter through town like children learning to skate—along with rushed celebrations. Snowballs are thrown, snowmen built. My friend Deborah dredged her closet and went cross-country skiing on the beach. Charming, yes. But how could spring dare to be late and then winter so fierce in this of all years? The garden was dormant. In local stores, fresh local produce was already reduced to root crops, garlic, onions, and that incredible survivor, tougher than any one of us, kale. I had run through internet lists of local farms, hoping for some new breakthrough. One, I noticed, promised olive oil. That was something we really had been missing. The farming family had a Greek name, so if anyone would know how to coax the trees along . . .

"No," the woman who answered the phone replied scornfully. "You can't grow olives here."

I hung up the phone, smiling inwardly. What would happen if we all stopped believing that so much is impossible? Only weeks ago I had spoken with a vineyard manager on nearby Saturna Island. His vines were arrayed on south-facing slopes wedged between the humid sea and a bank of rock walls that reflected the sun. The owners were thinking of putting in olive trees.

The future of local eating was looking better all the time.

"I learned how to smoke chum salmon," I said to James brightly, turning to face him in the bed. While visiting my mother's new home in the Cowichan Valley of Vancouver Island, I had met a Quw'utsun' man—that's how the native band spells the Anglicized word "Cowichan"—and the two of us started talking salmon. James and I had purchased five huge chum from Steve Johansen, who'd hooked them not even 10 miles from where we live, but I mentioned the fish humbly. Chum are sometimes called "dog salmon," in part because of their large, canine-like teeth but also because some Indian groups considered them best left to the dogs. Their flesh is a pale pink with only a hint of that classic salmon richness; the taste is closer to trout, but without the delicate lightness. The Quw'utsun' man, however, said that chum were very nice smoked.

James remained silent.

"You don't want to know how to smoke chum?" I said.

"Sure," he replied.

"We could do it in Dorreen," I said, beginning to count off the steps on my fingers. "First you gut the fish. Then you splay each one on a three-pronged stick. Then you hang them in a small smokehouse—the Quw'utsun' do thirty or forty at a time. Then you light an alderwood fire on the floor of the smokehouse and keep it going twenty-four hours a day for six or seven days—"

"That's it?" said James. "Just keep a fire burning twenty-four hours a day for a week?"

"We could do it in Dorreen," I said again, weakly this time.

"The bear would like that."

He did not seem to be himself these days. My mood had proved contagious. Meanwhile, I myself seemed to be seeing the world with different eyes. My mother's new home, for example: she had achieved the apotheosis of her water view. The cottage was still a rustic hodgepodge hung with tarps as she waited for the roofer to show, but from her living room picture window the Cowichan River was wide and glassy as it spilled from its headwaters lake. Forested hills kissed with mist rose on the opposite shore. A family of otters played on the dock; mergansers, widgeons, and wood ducks floated past. Yet my mother seemed unhappy with the place. It had been a last-minute choice. I hoped when the summer sun beamed on her vista—*Cowichan* means "warmed by the sun"—my mom would learn to love it. I found myself praying for her contentment, the same way I was suddenly hoping to penetrate James's cool distance.

Since our month in Dorreen, I'd been reading histories of that vast region cleft by the beautiful Skeena River. According to the Kitselas and Gitksan people who still live along its banks, the Skeena was once, probably thousands of years ago, home to a city called Dimlahamid. It is described as having been so large it took a crow a day to fly over it. For centuries on end, the people thrived on the bounty of the landscape. But finally the salmon no longer came and the forests were emptied of wildlife. The people of Dimlahamid were scattered.

"Great disasters are the landmarks of a people who are wise," says the Gitksan telling of the story. "They mark the ending of a time of error. They set a starting point for a better mode of life."

I had passed through my own time of errors, having failed to appreciate the bounty of my life. But there was still time to profit from the lesson. There had to be.

I would surprise James with a soup.

Of course, this was easier said than done. Cookbooks, with their insistent lists of nonlocal ingredients, were no use. All I had to guide me were mental images of James making soup, and vague memories of simple Japanese broths I had tasted. I was on my own, riffing.

Well, I knew a good place to start. I removed the tail portion of a chum salmon from the freezer. Frozen into blocks of ice, the chum was perfectly preserved—a trick we'd learned from the captain of the *Black Heart*—and we now knew, too, that salmon's flavor is strongest in the often-disdained tail. Next, I ransacked the fridge and cupboards. The options were seasonal, which is to say there wasn't much. The move to the balcony seemed to have arrested the decline of the onions, and I picked out one that was large and firm. I took down a dried hot pepper from the jacket closet. What caught my eye in the refrigerator was an immense celery root, an overlooked vegetable whose mild, tender flesh James had recently been serving raw. There is nothing handsome about celery root, also known as celeriac, with its octopus of rhizomes that no power-washing can completely clean, yet it was strangely appealing. Its oblong shape, its tuberous roots—it looks like a human heart. A pale, dirty human heart.

I would need a thickener, and set out to the grocery for kombu, a kind of kelp. I knew kombu from Japanese restaurants, and therefore had believed that it must grow exclusively on the islands of Japan and probably only on a patch of seaside rocks beneath the afternoon shadow of Mount Fuji, or something like that. In fact, the *Laminaria* genus occurs in temperate and arctic waters worldwide, and while *Laminaria japonica* is the classic kombu, *setchellii* is a comparable local species. It is collected on the open-ocean coast of Vancouver Island near the town of Bamfield, the richest seaweed ecology on earth and close to the limit of our 100-mile circle. The harvest is the most beautiful kind of agriculture, not even uprooting the plants from the seabed; rather, the kelp is mowed like a lawn.

Walking through the store I passed the usual temptations, from organic Ecuadorian bananas to French *sel de mer* to Mexican avocadoes, but my resolve was steeled not only by sheer will, but also by the fact that the 100-mile diet had by now developed enough notoriety that my picture had been splashed across newspaper pages and television screens. I had spoken at gatherings of local farmers, businesses, and foodies. Even at the till, I paused for only a second at the tantalizing sight of Denman Island dark chocolate. I suspect even saints were well behaved because they knew they were watched by higher powers.

Back home, after shaking the cold rain off my umbrella and hanging it on the front door handle to dry, I set to work in the kitchen. I spooned approximately one glob of butter into a large saucepan, set it on a burner, and turned to the onion. In the time it took me to peel it, I knew, James would have had the thing caramelized. I had to take the pot off the heat to avoid burning the butter as the onion's layers skidded out beneath my knife and I had to dice each slice individually. How did he do this day in and day out?

Grinding the chilies was easier, quick work with the hardwood mortar and pestle that was a gift from his father in distant Chile, where he had finally settled his wandering feet. I tossed the ruddy powder in with the onions and let the mixture fry until the kitchen filled with fumes that stung the eyes. Finally, I half-filled the pot with water, enjoying the first blast of steam as the liquid hit the molten oil, an effect I had observed many times but never by my own hand. There could be something to this cooking gig, after all.

When the water was boiling, I eased the heat and added the chum's tail and a large roll of kombu. Finally, I peeled the celery root, which proved surprisingly easy, chopped it into cubes, and heaped it into the mix. Almost instantly a smell filled the apartment. A good smell. After half an hour, I fished out the large lump of salmon. The skin pulled away easily, and the meat came off the bones with a minimum of effort. I broke the fillet into flakes and returned it to the pot. Suddenly it looked like soup. It really did. The broth was pale brown with just enough thickness to glaze the dense chunks of celery root and chum, each tender to the fork. I brought the boil to the barest simmer and set the table with two glasses of white wine.

James came in the front door, which looks straight down a short hallway into the kitchen.

"I made dinner," I said casually.

Famously unflappable, he managed not to appear surprised. "What's cooking?" he said.

"It's ready," I replied. "Come to the table."

He did appear to be moving in slow motion, maybe buying time to process this strange new occurrence. He stood with the door open for a minute, as though he might need to escape. Instead he came down the hall and passed through the kitchen, where he paused to touch my hip and look me in the eye. Then he took the seat farthest from the stove—the one seat he never sits in. I placed one steaming bowl in front of him, and sat down across the table. I watched his face as he blew on the spoon. At last he smiled, the first taste of dinner still suspended in front of his mouth.

"I never thought I'd live to see you make a soup," he said.

"But is it good?" I asked.

He put the spoon in his mouth and closed his eyes, looking for a moment like a child asleep.

"It's good," he said, his eyes now wide and blue with wonder. "It's a very good chum soup."

"You would not have been *my* good chum if you'd said anything else."

I could call it beginner's luck, but of course it was more than that. I had not moved effortlessly through the kitchen, the way he does, with even four courses seeming to fall into time with one another. I had bumped both elbows and scalded a finger. Mine was the simplest soup, but I had put so much into it. This dinner was different from those I had cooked in my times alone; it had the flavor of the dishes that James had made for me every day of our lives together.

Outside it was snowing again, big, wet flakes that stuck to the dining nook window. Christmas was coming, but this was the meal we'd remember. Two people wrapped in a cloud of steam that only we could share.

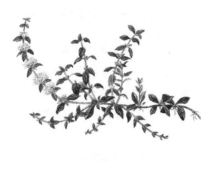

→✳ 100-MILE SANGRIA BLANCA ✳←

1 BOTTLE WHITE WINE

1 $\frac{1}{2}$ CUPS HIGHBUSH CRANBERRIES

3 CUPS FROZEN BLUEBERRIES

2 CUPS HARD APPLE CIDER

POUR WINE OVER BERRIES IN A LARGE PUNCH BOWL. LET SIT COVERED FOR 24 HOURS. CHILL. USING A SLOTTED SPOON, REMOVE MOST BERRIES, LEAVING SOME FOR PRESENTATION. ADD APPLE CIDER JUST BEFORE SERVING TO MAINTAIN EFFERVESCENCE. GARNISH EACH GLASS WITH ADDITIONAL FROZEN BLUEBERRIES.

JANUARY

MAKE SOIL, NOT WAR.

GRAFFITI

The New Year's Eve party scene was not an option. Yes, it was true that we had sneaked a canapé or two at holiday parties, feeling the shaming eyes of the world and shushing each other, *"Don't tell the internet."* Still, failing to turn down quality shortbread is a far cry from entirely giving in to a New Year's extravaganza with champagne all night from France, Spain, and California, and a nosh table covered in tropical fruit. We needed a different way to turn the calendar on a year of local eating. We would stay home. We would sit in our little apartment and eat the good products of the good earth, and we would not sin.

Anyway, I had a cold.

I suspected we could drag Ruben and Olive into our born-to-be-mild evening, on account of their recently developed Theory of the Pirogi Party. In November they had attended a get-together hosted by a self-declared "Pirogi King" of Polish descent in order to stuff a small mountain of the traditional dumplings. After each step in the process the Pirogi King would lead the masses in a Polish folksong followed by a shot of vodka. Making pirogi involves many steps, as it turns out, and the feast at night's end was an unsteady blur of laughter, camaraderie, and, for some, eventual nausea. The following day, Ruben declared his hypothesis: that a night making food with friends will *always* be a more worthwhile experience than, say, watching a blockbuster movie. Olive had tested the concept with a surprise pirogi-making party for Ruben's birthday in early December. I brought along a filling of homemade sauerkraut and Fraser Valley mushrooms, along with a bottle of local wine and a certain skepticism. The sense of community was slow to build. Almost everyone in attendance was an industrial designer, and much of the night was dedicated to a fierce critique of Hunky Bill's pirogi maker, a Vancouver invention that, like many labor-saving devices, significantly slowed our progress. By some silent consensus, "the device" was finally abandoned in favor of making each pirogi by hand, and the roomful of emphatic individuals was freed to express itself. Within half an hour, two Québécoises were leading us in French drinking songs and everyone was head-to-toe in flour. Nothing memorable was said, but it was all very funny.

The Theory of the Pirogi Party seemed to hold. And Ruben and Olive would not be able to forgo a 100-mile dinner to attend some glitzy commercial spectacle involving fireworks, burlesque girls, and Cuban cigars.

I had decided to make pasta, the one wheat-product craving Alisa and I had yet to satisfy. Alisa had found a hand-cranked Italian pasta maker in a thrift store for twenty dollars. It appeared to work. I had never made pasta from scratch before, but then I'd never made sauerkraut, pickles, crackers, jelly, or so many other things before this year. I'd never stayed in on New Year's Eve, either.

"I'm too sick for this," I said.

Alisa filled my glass with cyser. The gesture was bittersweet; for the first time since childhood, there would be no champagne to toast the old year and cheer the new. Alisa had called every winery within 100 miles and, yes, several of them produce sparkling wines, and yes, we were too late to reserve a bottle. "But I *love* champagne," she'd said—she has been known to celebrate events as humble as laundry day with a flute or two of bubbly—and now she had to accept the hard fact that this year's celebration would strictly involve wine and cider.

I kneaded the pasta dough, pounding out the past year's abundant troubles, while Alisa wrestled with a blueberry pie. Outside, a squall attacked the windows; I let the dough rest and pressed my hot forehead against the glass. I would make a simple tomato sauce. Not everything in a life needs to be difficult. We had agreed, too, that for first-time pasta chefs, fettuccine noodles would be safest—wide enough that they might actually hold together. But this was New Year's Eve, I thought as I rolled balls of dough into flat sheets. The night demanded risk.

"I'm putting it through the spaghetti roller," I said defiantly.

"You'll only regret it," said Alisa. "Be cautious."

"Spaghetti," I said firmly.

Her argument was cut short as beautiful tresses of spaghetti reeled out of the pasta maker, and it took both of us, side by side, to carry the noodles, laid across our forearms, to the kitchen table. Then I was rolling more dough, cranking more noodles, oven doors slamming, pots boiling over, the room filling with timeless smells, Ruben and Olive arriving in the midst of it all with a tub of homemade, 100-mile *labna*—yogurt cheese—and enough cyser to refill our glasses. We sat down with loaded plates.

"It's hard to express how excited I am at having made pasta," I said.

We dug in. The noodles were nutty, creamy, comforting, an antidote to the weather that knocked over garbage cans in the quiet streets. We had retired to the couches when two more friends appeared, surprise visitors dropping in with best wishes between parties. But we fed them pie, and homemade crackers with cheese, and our whole month's pickle ration, and plenty of wine and cyser, and then it was time to count down the minutes. We turned to the clock. It is a nineteenth-century French black marble mantel clock that Alisa had inherited from her grandfather and insisted be put on display, despite the fact that in a shoebox apartment it looks like a cheap imposter. Yet this was its moment. It chimed midnight with unquestionable nobility, and Alisa and I stole the New Year's first kiss with smiling lips.

Then our friends brought out a certain bottle, from Spain, and we decided that the powers that decide these things must have wanted us to have champagne after all.

Rain. The January rains are the cruelest, spilling unbroken through the bare branches of the trees. Even the densest evergreens are saturated, and beneath them the drops fall long and hard after the storm itself has passed. It is cold rain, too, nearly sleet, and it finds its way behind the ears and down the crease of the spine. The truly serious rains began in earnest on December 19, and radio forecasters soon started to wonder aloud whether the city might break the standing record of twenty-eight consecutive rainy days, set in 1953. These are our monsoons, and it seems almost shameful that there isn't a local name.

Rain reduces the world. A few blocks seem like too far to go, and 100 miles unimaginably distant. Why leave the apartment? For that matter, why get out of bed? A person can get a lot done in bed. Though the sound of the rain outside is soothing . . .

"How do you feel?" asked Alisa one morning in the first days of January. I had my feet thrust out from the covers, my morning ritual to cool down after a night under the crushing blanket that Alisa insists on for winter. Her question seemed to be referring to my health.

"How do *you* feel?" I replied.

"I asked you first."

"You asked me first because you were worried about something yourself," I parlayed, and she conceded with a smile.

"I feel fine, I think."

"I think I feel fine, too."

"No, but—*good,* actually," she said.

I had a sense of what she was attempting to communicate. I had noticed, for example, that my meals had grown steadily smaller and simpler. For breakfast, a slice of Alisa's home-baked bread plus a single boiled egg dusted with dried bull kelp and hot pepper flakes, and a snifter of frozen blueberries. Or, for dinner, a salad of chopped red cabbage, walnuts, apple, and potato alongside a trio of raw oysters, with applesauce for dessert. Each ingredient was bold and didn't need a lot of fancy cooking, but, more important, the food seemed to go straight to my blood and my brain. I rarely felt hungry, and whatever cravings I did have came through with hair-splitting clarity. I might suddenly want exactly one slice of cheese, or red kuri squash—no other squash would do—for lunch. I was having a peculiarly electric conversation with my body about its needs. It felt cosmic, and therefore embarrassing.

Still, we wondered. Most of what we now ate had been in storage for weeks if not months in cupboards, the freezer, or jars; meanwhile, everyone around us was buying long-distance sunshine in the form of mangoes and mandarin oranges. It was Alisa who brought up the word *scurvy,* the largely forgotten vitamin C deficiency that once plagued European sailing-ship crews on their long ocean crossings. I countered with the fact that the Dietary Reference Intakes—the daily nutrition guidelines developed by the Washington, D.C.–based National Academy of Sciences—offer a list of "selected food sources" for vitamin C. Tomatoes, tomato juice, Brussels sprouts, cauliflower, strawberries, cabbage, and spinach are on the list. So are potatoes. The only two selected sources we weren't regularly eating were citrus fruits and broccoli.

I was more worried about protein. We had eggs and dairy products; walnuts, a few chestnuts, and—for me—hazelnuts; as well as a limited supply of fava, green soy, black, and pinto beans picked up from the region's more experimental farmers. Shellfish taste like a clean sea breeze in the colder months, in much the same way that carrots and beets are better after they've been touched by a frost, and winter fish are richer in savory oils. Unfortunately, fish from the Salish Sea remained notable by their absence. The last had been the sardines. I hadn't known there were sardines in the Pacific Ocean. They have to be fresh—the freshest. Grab a sardine in your fist by the tail and hold the head upright at twelve o'clock. Does the fish flop down to six o'clock? Forget it. Any farther than three o'clock and that fish is past its prime. In any case, the sardines had vanished from the fish shops a month ago.

We were holing up. The few restaurant visits we'd allowed ourselves under our 100-mile rules had been abandoned as we immersed ourselves ever deeper in the experiment. Even the supermarket had become unfamiliar, and if we did pay a visit, our shopping list had a nostalgic simplicity: a bottle of milk, a pound of butter, a block of cheese. We could pull our grocery budget out of the bowl that held our spare change. It was winter outside, but summertime in the freezer, where I could dig for the peas, green beans, red currants, prawns, and so on that we'd put away months ago. Our diet no longer felt "different." It had become the new normal. At least that was the view from within the white walls of our apartment.

Then came the call to have dinner with the critics.

The Raincity Grill is a high-end Pacific Northwest restaurant, one of the most committed of those that have emerged over the past two decades in the region. The chef, Andrea Carlson, is among the growing list of master cooks who advocate for the fresh and local, but she had never taken the step to an entirely local provenance. Now she was planning a 100-mile tasting menu. And could we come to a trial dinner or two?

We took the bus to the most beautiful part of downtown,

English Bay, where the mid-January sunset was nothing more than a shading of slate into black. By some miraculous alignment of the planets, the neighborhood had never ceded to the boringly rich. English Bay remains a place where you might meet minor Russian mobsters, honeymooning gay men, Korean exchange students, elderly couples who complain about the pace of change but wouldn't move if you offered them Buckingham Palace. The variety fades when you step beneath the eaves of Raincity Grill, but not by so much. It's a day's-wages restaurant, while many others can cost a whole week of your life, and its candlelight is a bulwark against the chill and the damp.

The food critics were waiting. Their faces hovered over a long table. In specific, they awaited the Redonda Island oyster pannacotta with Dungeness crab leg and Agassiz coho roe cured with epazote (the herb formerly known as "wormseed"). To start.

"Exactly the kind of thing we eat all the time," I said, in answer to the obvious question. Scanning the other five courses, I made a mental note never again to serve "goat cheese" in my house. From now on, it was *chèvre.*

As we ran through the evening's menu—Cortes Island honey mussels, Agassiz chestnut gnocchi sauté—the food critics slouched attentively, the way owls ear for mice. This was the opposite of the Pirogi Party: here was a meal in which none of us at the table had participated, and yet over which we stood in judgment. It was the modern way of eating, food as a miracle that appears on the plate, immaculately conceived. On the other hand, Andrea Carlson was very much a real person, shy enough that she would only face us later, slightly hidden by a goblet of wine. She was nonetheless able to stand her ground alone as an artist, and was the only one among us armed with a brace of enormous knives.

We reached the braised lamb neck (which Alisa and I would sidestep) with Hyslop crab apples and roasted sunchokes. The sommelier, who was every inch a sommelier, leaned into the table. The red table wine he was about to serve, he said, was produced on Salt Spring Island, but the grapes had come from the Okanagan Valley, nearly 200 miles away. "We just couldn't find a local red that had the strengths to pair with lamb."

Out of nowhere, here was the Big Question, the ultimate conundrum of the 100-mile diet and every other exercise that might stray from the path of least resistance. *Why bother?* There was a bottle of good red wine on the table. Did we have to turn it into something complicated?

For Alisa and me, the answer was no longer a simple sound bite. Even the ugly statistic—at least 1,500 miles from farm to plate for the typical food item in North America—had proved to be only a gateway into a deeper problem. In fact, the simple concept of food miles is an easy target. Seeing a movement toward local food in the United Kingdom, the Agribusiness and Economics Research Unit of Lincoln University in New Zealand studied the total amount of energy used to bring apples, onions, dairy products, and sheep's meat to market in Britain versus the same products shipped 11,000 miles from New Zealand. The researchers found that, owing to the heavy energy consumption of industrial farming in the U.K., it was actually *more efficient* to maintain the $330 million trade from New Zealand than to have the British raise these products on their own. Of course, the study's findings also make an unspoken argument for a different way forward: farm more efficiently in Britain. In 2005 a team of academics from the University of Essex and London's City University estimated the environmental price tag of U.K. farming at £1.51 billion. A switch to strictly organic production, the study found, could reduce those costs by 75 percent.

Meanwhile, the long table of food critics fell silent. Alisa and I, trying to be agreeable about the red wine, murmured supportive nostrums.

A voice piped up.

"So there is one item on the 100-Mile Menu that is *not* from within 100 miles?"

The publicist flushed, tastefully, and there was some hemming and hawing about the quality of certain kinds of Fraser Valley grape.

I had expected the 100-mile experiment to be a platform to think about many things, among them a long list of bummers from climate change to the failure of whole generations to learn how to recognize edible mushrooms. What I could see around the table now was a less tangible consideration: a sense of adventure. We are at a point in world history where bad news about the state of the Earth is just as jaded and timeworn as the idea that there is nowhere left to go, nothing new to explore. Put those two statements side by side, however, and something hidden is revealed. Of course there are new things to do, and no shortage of them. We need to find new ways to live into the future. We can start anytime; we can live them here and now. The food critics didn't want to reduce this local dinner to a question of mileage. But neither did they want to cover up the meal's weaknesses and challenges, its element of the unexpected. They wanted to explore the intersection of reality and possibility.

"I think you might revisit that wine selection," said one of the food critics.

"You cannot have a 100-Mile Menu that fails to draw from within 100 miles," said another quite reasonably.

The offending wine, and with it the lamb, were stricken from the menu by popular demand.

There was beef in the freezer. The flesh of a dead cow. It had been there a few weeks before I learned that Alisa had bought the packets—stewing meat and ground beef—on a whim that she couldn't explain even to herself. She had listened to her instincts. Perhaps she knew that the meat's time was bound to come.

I put a pound on the counter. For the first time in eighteen years I was cooking with red meat, but the moment didn't feel particularly sacred. For nearly two decades the idea hadn't been acceptable to me, and now, this day, it was. While disease scares and product recalls were making more and more people fearful of their food, Alisa and I were moving in the opposite direction. We were effectively off the industrial grid, eating from now-trusted producers whose standards we could question face-to-face. Any outbreak of disease—always a possibility—was likely to be contained by the farms' small scale and easy traceability. Our faith in the food we were eating was higher than ever before; in fact, we'd only realized how much confidence we'd lost in the food system when we started to regain it.

I could not, in any case, claim that I was still a vegetarian. For months now, I had feasted on seafood and dairy. Throughout history, human beings who have relied on this North Pacific landscape have killed and eaten animals as an ecological necessity. Our 100-mile diet had taken Alisa and me to that point. I felt respect for the flesh of the cow, but by now it wouldn't matter if it had been a garlic clove or a pole bean instead. I had seen the way a garlic stalk gathers the rain like a spiral fountain and delivers it down to its roots; the way autumn bean pods furl into tight, dry ringlets, literally ejecting the seed. I had learned to be awestruck by living things.

I heated some butter in a frying pan, and the cold meat crackled against the oil. When the fat had cooked out of the meat I poured it off, leaving just enough grease to sauté a sliced onion. I bruised some rosemary with the pestle and threw in a handful, and now the odors seemed to take me back as far as the discovery of fire.

So I would eat meat tonight. Not so much had changed. Out there in the wider world, beyond the inward-turning 100-mile experiment, it was still the norm that farm animals suffered lives that few of us could witness and still stomach the meat at the end of our forks. I could. The cow I was about to eat had been raised according to the "biodynamic" principles first proposed in 1924 by the Austrian philosopher Rudolf Steiner, who imagined farms as entities operating in accord with natural processes. The cow had been conceived through actual sex, rather than by artificial insemination, and, as a calf, was reared with other calves for company. It nursed from its mother, then ate grass or, in winter, organic hay. Its horns were never removed. The adult cow ranged freely or took shelter according to its innate behavior, and its manure became a part of the farm cycle. Never in its life did it feel an electric goad, and on slaughtering day, the following principle was applied: "One should be conscious of the fact that the death of a living being with a soul precedes all meat processing." Over the past months I'd met a farmer who holds her chickens until their heartbeats slow before swiftly killing them; I'd heard about a man who burns sage to honor his lambs and then slaughters them in their sleep. In the Burgoyne Valley of Salt Spring Island, I spent some time with George Laundry, a former physicist in his sixties who, to go lightly on the land, allows himself just twenty gallons of diesel fuel per year for his tractor and does everything else by hand. A neighboring farmer, Laundry said, refuses even to break the soil. He simply casts out seeds and reaps whatever comes.

These are degrees of eccentricity, I suppose, or what we might otherwise call mysticism. I suspect, too, that they are reactions to the soul-shock of modern life with all its cold separation and routine violence, and not so different, perhaps, from the decision to eat close to home for a year. With our regular sojourns into the fields surrounding Vancouver, Alisa and I had seen the relentless advance of the city. The change had always seemed sad in the way that any loss of innocence is sad, but now it seemed like lunacy, impossibly wrongheaded. According to the U.S. Department of Agriculture and the American Farmland Trust, the United States throughout the 1990s lost more than two acres of agricultural land to development every minute. In Canada, where only 5 percent of the land base is classified as "dependable" for agriculture, cities now cover 50 percent more farmland than they did thirty years ago. The conversion is a fundamentalist act—a pattern that assumes we have been liberated forever from the need to live in a real place, in real time.

Seen with 100-mile eyes, the global supermarket offered nothing for the cold, wet months. Laundry, on the other hand, once grew twenty-one different organic winter crops on his handful of acres. We missed pancake syrup; a forester named Gary Backlund introduced us to the fact that syrup could be—and was being—made from the sap of the local bigleaf maple, a fragment of knowledge that was better known in the nineteenth century than it is today. At the beginning of the new millennium, the World Bank reported that 43 percent of the world's arable land was already degraded to some degree; but there was a time when human beings drew their food from every conceivable environment, from the desert to the arctic ice pack. Every inch of the planet can sustain us. It only needs to be restored.

I took the meat and onions off the heat, let them cool a few minutes, then dusted the mixture with flour until everything was well coated. Some potatoes were simmering; I stirred their cooking water into the pan, then poured everything into the soup pot. Finally, I took a spoonful. It tasted like my old memories of beef stew. Well, it needed a little salt. That damnable salt from Oregon.

The water still fell from the sky in buckets, in sheets, in tantrums. Friends, relatives, even news reporters looked out their windows on the bleak northern landscape and then picked up their telephones. They had a question for Alisa and me.

"How do you feel?"

We felt fine, thank you.

I would eventually place a call to the Tampa, Florida, home of Cynthia Sass, a registered dietician and spokesperson for the American Dietetics Association on, among other things, environmental nutrition. Almost immediately she mentioned that she had just purchased a bag of Florida avocados, which I instantly desired though I hadn't thought of them in weeks. As it turned out, Sass had heard about our year of eating locally. And would she, as a dietician, recommend such a diet to the average American?

She laughed in a way that suggested she was rolling her eyes, then managed to say, "Yes, I would."

As many have begun to realize, the question—*how do you feel?*—is best turned on mainstream North America itself. According to consumption statistics for ground beef and frozen potatoes, the average U.S. citizen eats the equivalent of three hamburgers and four orders of fries a week. That same typical American drinks more than twice as much soda as milk. In 2004, Gladys Block, a professor of epidemiology and nutrition at the University of California, Berkeley, completed an analysis of the U.S. National Health and Nutrition Examination Survey, which is possibly the most comprehensive examination of eating habits carried out in any nation. Block found that sweets, soft drinks, and alcoholic beverages accounted for almost 25 percent of all calories consumed in America. Add in salty snacks and fruity drinks, and the total reaches one-third of calorie intake. Meanwhile, Americans eat half as many servings of vegetables as recommended; 50 percent of the vegetables they *do* eat comprise just three foods: iceberg lettuce, potatoes, and canned tomatoes.

Food begins to lose nutrition as soon as it is harvested. Fruit and vegetables that travel shorter distances are therefore likely to be closer to a maximum of nutrition. "Nowadays, we know a lot more about the naturally occurring substances in produce," said Sass. "It's not just vitamins and minerals, but all these phytochemicals and really powerful disease-fighting substances, and we do know that when a food never really reaches its peak ripeness, the levels of these substances never get as high."

The principle extends to stored foods. For healthy eating, Sass recommends that people do exactly what Alisa and I had done: gather fresh foods at their peak, freeze or can the surplus, and consume them within six months. "You haven't got *exactly* the same nutrition," she said, "but actually it's pretty darn close." As an added bonus, foods processed at home won't contain the long rap sheet of unpronounceable additives that appear in super-market versions of foods as simple as pasta sauce, biscuits, or popcorn. Seasonality, too, is good for our bodies, said Sass. North Americans typically eat a set of familiar foods year-round; eating with the changing seasons actually forces them out of their habits. "We always talk about eating the rainbow of colors. The pigments that give purple cabbage its color have different phyto-chemicals than what would be in, say, a white family vegetable like garlic or leeks or onions," said Sass. "Even people who tend to eat healthier still get into that rut of eating the same foods all the time."

Sass teaches at the University of South Florida, and each year canvasses her students to find out what foods they have *never* eaten. She is astounded by the list: fresh berries and cherries, kiwi fruit, apricots, rhubarb, and plums; arugula, Swiss chard, kale, beets, artichokes, and rutabaga. "It really is sad, because going to the farmers' market was one of my favorite all-time memories of being a kid, and having a garden, and doing all the things that my mother would let me do in the kitchen—making fresh pies, making homemade applesauce, homemade ice cream. All these things that we grew or got at the farmers' markets, I meet a lot of kids who've never seen these things growing. They've only seen them at the store."

Yet when I called to confirm these facts with Marion Nestle, a professor and former chair of nutrition, food studies, and public health at New York University, she waved away the nutrition issue as a red herring. Yes, she said, our 100-mile diet—even in winter—was almost certainly more nutritious than what the average American was eating. That doesn't mean it is *necessary* to eat locally in order to be healthy. In fact, a person making smart choices from the global megamart can easily meet all the body's needs.

"There will be nutritional differences, but they'll be marginal," said Nestle. "I mean, that's not really the issue. It *feels* like it's the issue—obviously fresher foods that are grown on better soils are going to have more nutrients. But people are not nutrient-deprived. We're just not nutrient-deprived."

So would Marion Nestle, as a dietician, as one of America's most important critics of dietary policy, advocate for local eating?

"Absolutely."

Why? Because she loves the taste of fresh food, she said. She loves the mystery of years when the late corn is just utterly, incredibly good, and no one can say why: it just is. She likes having farmers around, and farms, and farmland. I thought back to the meal I had eaten on New Year's Eve. It was so much more than "local food." The crackers brought to mind Hamish Crawford in his wheat field, and our friend Adrienne driving through a blizzard to pick up our three pails of flour. The noodles recalled the rise and fall of wheat farming in the Pacific Northwest. The sauce was an autumn afternoon gleaning tomatoes with Alisa, and I could now look back and smile at how we'd bickered while we canned. I'd spiced the sauce with coriander from Vancouver Island; bay leaf from the community garden; oregano from the balcony pots; onions from the farmers' market; garlic from an old comrade; ground walnuts purchased in the fog alongside my prodigal brother. The labna cheese: a moment of Rubenesque inspiration. The smell of blueberries from the oven: a spring day, when everything was new. It wasn't a meal; it was a memoir. We had become a part of the story of our food.

"We have an insane food system, one that's totally based on cheap oil," said Nestle. Is it possible to build a new and different system closer to home? It is. The lesser economies of scale could be partially offset by greater employment on small farms. Subsidies, like the $20,000 the U.S. government spends on every corn grower each year, could support that small-farm economy rather than factory operations and industrial monocultures. Any of this is possible, and more. "But it's theoretical. Is it possible to do it in practice? That's politics. People have to demand it and exercise their democratic rights."

As January ended, the rain still fell.

→✳ THE LAST COURSE ✳←

$\frac{1}{4}$ CUP HONEY

1 $\frac{1}{2}$ CUPS WARM WATER

$\frac{1}{2}$ CUP FROZEN RHUBARB

$\frac{1}{2}$ LB MEDIUM-FIRM CHEESE, E.G., TOMME

$\frac{1}{2}$ CUP WALNUTS, ROASTED AND CRUSHED

ADD HONEY, WATER, AND RHUBARB TO A SAUCEPAN OVER MEDIUM HEAT. BRING TO A BOIL, THEN REDUCE HEAT AND SIMMER, STIRRING OCCASIONALLY, UNTIL THE RHUBARB COMES APART AND ABOUT $\frac{1}{2}$ CUP OF LIQUID REMAINS. PREHEAT OVEN TO 250°F. SLICE CHEESE INTO SERVING-SIZE TRIANGLES AND ARRANGE ON A PLATE. WARM IN OVEN UNTIL JUST SLUMPING. PLACE EACH CHEESE SLICE ON AN INDIVIDUAL SMALL PLATE. DRIZZLE RHUBARB-HONEY REDUCTION OVER TOP THROUGH A STRAINER. GARNISH WITH WALNUTS AND ENJOY THE LAST LONG NIGHTS OF THE YEAR.

FEBRUARY

WE BELIEVE THAT THIS WORLD WOULD BE HAPPIER
IF IT HAD MORE GOOD PLAIN COOKS.

THE GOOD HOUSEKEEPING COOK BOOK

We were looking at the snow—it was a mess. Sunny Johnson, a pretty twenty-eight-year-old with high cheekbones and killing hands who lived in the Minnesota pine country, was standing in front of her garage to pose for a photograph.

"That on the snow. That's still the blood from where I killed a rooster last fall. First rooster I ever killed."

I looked uneasily at the dark patches. "That must have been hard for you," I said.

"No, not all," she said vehemently, almost with glee. "It was easy. I'd do it again."

I'd been zooming in on her face, but panned out again to take in the blood. It seemed to represent something—the raw core of self-sufficiency, perhaps, which I respected but wasn't sure I could approach.

But that was a personal question. As the idea of our 100-mile diet had traveled, I had heard it said that James and I had it easy

233

living in the Pacific Northwest. Forget the fact that we were at 49 degrees north latitude, where the winter solstice sees only eight hours of daylight and the average annual rainfall is a comfortable swimming depth—eating locally on the West Coast was apparently no great challenge. On the other hand, eating locally was "impossible"—the word was often used by these critics—in places where the winter was long and cold, which seemed to be anywhere but where we lived, including the Deep South. So: I was here at the frozen headwaters of the Mississippi River. I had asked Sunny to open her kitchen and, by extension, her life to me.

She was game. Sunny and two of her friends, Steve Dahlberg and Stephanie Williams, teach at the White Earth Tribal and Community College in Mahnomen, Minnesota. They were also the core of a one-year local eating experiment with parallels to our own. Wiser than James and I, their seven-person group had launched in September, having foraged and preserved foods all summer to prepare. They allowed themselves a 250-mile radius, and tried to make wild foods a significant part of their diet. I felt hapless in comparison. These were the kind of people who could survive in the wilderness with just the clothes on their backs and a knife; Steve even made his own knife. What I learned from these folks wouldn't necessarily translate into my urban life—to begin with, packing a blade in the city sends a totally different message. The lessons of Minnesota, however, might just turn the "impossible" into the thoroughly real.

We took off down snowy roads in Sunny's dark green pickup. Her toddler Saelyn, whose father was a Navajo from the Four Corners reservation in the Southwest, played intently with plastic cowboys on the seat between us. When his mother stopped the truck to point to the sky—"An eagle!" she exclaimed—he looked up and murmured, "My friend, my friend." Sunny was clearly rapt at the sight of the threatened American icon; I didn't have the heart to tell her I saw bald eagles often. Still, I associated them so strongly with the sea that I was amazed to see one soaring over a frozen river in the heart of the continent. As the bird became a dot in the far distance, we continued on our way, Sunny tugging open paper bags and beginning to explain some of her food sources.

"This is wintergreen"—the dried leaf was bitter on my tongue—"you can make a tea from it, or soak it in alcohol to make a liniment for sore joints. Those are rose hips"—and she pulled the truck to the shoulder, leaping out to pick an orange bulb from a roadside shrub. It was bland and pulpy. "It's got lots of vitamin C, and it makes a great jelly," Sunny enthused. We carried on. "Milkweed is a wonderful, versatile plant. You can eat the shoots in the spring like asparagus. The flower heads are like broccoli. And I like to clean out the pods—inside is a cheese alternative." It sounded intriguing, but I wasn't necessarily sure it would catch on.

Sunny's kitchen was crammed with slightly more conventional, savory foods. For our dinner she fried up buffalo burgers with a side of wild rice for a real taste of Minnesota. "It's so nice to meet someone who has the same values I do—but doesn't think the world is coming to an end," she said as we confided life stories over a bottle of Domaine de Chaberton. I had, for perhaps the first time since Prohibition, smuggled our heavily taxed Canadian booze *into* America at the obscure border crossing between Tolstoi, Manitoba, and Lancaster, Minnesota. Anyone in Sunny's experiment was allowed a dozen "trade items" from anywhere on earth, which they could share if members of the group ate together; Sunny had cleverly included alcohol on her list. Others went with chocolate, potato chips, yeast, salt, even bottled water and hominy grits.

"Your friends think the world is going to end?" I said as we sat by the woodstove in her cozy living room; hers was a proud hippie house, built halfway into a hillside by the original owners. The roof was sown with wildflowers and weeds allowed to run riot, though the squirrels, she acknowledged, were hell.

"It's in the Mayan prophecies."

"That would be depressing," I said, nodding wisely and pretending I knew what she was talking about. The popular interpretation, it seems, has the world ending on December 22, 2012. Why eat locally at all? Why not wear Florida panther coats and drive racing cars along the edges of cliffs? I'd have to ask them about it later.

Sunny's parents were back-to-the-landers. Her father, the son of a CIA spy, had rejected his family's straitlaced values to hitchhike across America; his beatnik travels landed him in Minnesota, where he fell in love with a local girl. They raised Sunny on 160 acres with no electricity or running water. It was a lonely experience for an only child, she said, but she was clearly heir to her family's self-sufficient ideals.

The following morning was Sunny's wild-foods class, and she gave me a tour of the small college building. In the classroom, Steve and Stephanie sat at tables in what usually served as a science lab, with microscopes and test tubes all around. A handful of students, about half of them from the Anishinabe reservation, lounged in running shoes, T-shirts, one guy even in shorts. Apparently I was the only one unaware that the class van had broken down and we were not going into the bush. I felt ridiculously overdressed in my winter boots and gaiters.

"Well, some people are missing, and there are some new faces here," said Steve, "but I guess we'll begin with what we've got." A few more students wandered in as the lesson in how to identify local trees progressed. By the time we started trooping around outside, I appreciated my boots; it had been one of the warmest Januarys on record in the Midwest, and the outside world was ankle-deep slush. I was out of my element—terrible at identifying Minnesota's trees. Even the sullen teenager in striped warm-up pants did better.

I asked Steve, who looked very Average Joe in his jeans and eyeglasses, what had brought him to his extreme of local eating. "I was already eating lots of local food," he said. "I grew up on a little farm near here. I'd rather they got a bigger piece of the action than the suits in the city." He liked plain food eaten in season, he said. He didn't like bananas and he didn't need salad in winter.

And what about the end of the world? He wasn't hitching his wagon to that 2012 date, he said, but his doctoral studies in global warming convinced him some big changes were going down. His North Dakota homestead skills would be absolutely crucial. The end of society as we know it wouldn't necessarily be a bad thing, he said. "Even if it turns out to be some perfect-world utopia, it's still better to eat local foods. It just makes life better!" I appreciated his peppy view of Armageddon.

One of Steve's big hobbies was fermenting, well, anything edible. I was dimly aware that this method of preserving food had developed a sort of cult following since the 2003 publication of *Wild Fermentation: The Flavor, Nutrition, and Craft of Live-Culture Foods,* by a former New York City policy wonk named Sandor Ellix Katz. In fact, James had used—and continued to use—the author's sauerkraut recipe to odorize our apartment. Properly prepared fermented foods contain "probiotics," or living bacteria that can help improve or maintain the microecology of the human digestive tract. Certainly the majority of the world's cuisines include far more fermented products than ours in mainstream North America, from French blue cheese to Japanese miso to Iceland's more challenging *hákarl*—putrefied Greenland shark. "Whatever doesn't kill you makes you fatter," said Steve, and laughed.

Stephanie rolled her eyes. "I don't like all that fermented stuff. But local food is how I was raised." She'd grown up on "the rez," and wore a jacket embroidered with POWWOW COMMITTEE. With the exception of flour and sugar, said Stephanie, "I never ate food from a grocery store until I was a teenager." Their food supplies were hunted game and vegetables from the family garden. But she had fallen into new habits; she'd been addicted to soda for the last five years, and didn't want to set a bad example for her kids. "Now, everyone here knows about what I'm doing. They look in my grocery cart at the store, and I'm held accountable."

Stephanie and Sunny had traveled the West on their motorcycles going to wild-food conferences, but had grown tired of the academic approach. "People would talk about, 'Maybe we should look for funding to design a study to see what people

think about local eating?' " Stephanie recalled. "Finally we just
said, 'Enough talking, let's do it.' "

"I'm not an evangelist," said Steve. "But lots of people are on
the verge, and we can be a trigger."

As the class ended, Steve invited me to try some of his fermentation experiments. He led me to their office's small kitchen.
"Here's some plums," he said, taking out a jar. I popped a dark
purple orb the size of a marble into my mouth. It fizzed across my
tongue, and it was everything I could do to keep from spitting it
out. "Mmm," I said, trying to look as if I were enjoying it.

"I really love those," said Becky, a chatty, middle-aged woman
with orange corkscrew hair who had followed us from the classroom. "Want to see my mushroom tea?" She pulled out a jar
with shaggy fungus in a muddy brown liquid.

"You drink that?" I asked. I was incredibly relieved when she
didn't ask me to try it. Next, Steve said, he wanted to make a
traditional local drink from fermented beets, a recipe handed
down by the descendents of Minnesota's many Eastern European
and Russian settlers. *Kvass.* The word sounded like an insult. *It
tastes like your kvass.*

But every region on earth has its more unique foods (the Pacific Northwest tribes prized their decomposed oolichan grease),
along with its comforts and pleasures. I was excited about Minnesota wild rice. "Ricing" is a verb in the state, and "the size of a
rice stick" is a familiar unit of measurement. Sunny drove me to
the house of her local supplier. He had a large canvas teepee
painted with what looked like a crab in his front yard, as well as
a large chunk of meat hanging on the front porch, in cold storage
as it were. I bought five pounds of wild rice, and he threw in a

large bag of broken grains for free. With butter and brown sugar, he said, they made a delicious porridge. I paid twenty-five dollars for a haul that would have cost me more than twice as much at home.

Back in Sunny's kitchen, it was somehow surprising to see the same foods tucked away as on our shelves in Vancouver: dried chili peppers, braids of garlic, rows of squash. No, all was not a struggle in midwinter Minnesota; in fact, eating locally here was in many ways easier than at home. Sunny's pantry was lined with jars of locally milled white and rye flour, as well as pearl barley and white sugar from sugar beets. A transplanted Frenchman helped brew red-wine vinegar, not to mention cook up pâtés and sausages. It had taken her three months to find supplies of dried beans, but Sunny now had more than she knew what to do with. She put some in bags for me to take home: black, pinto, and kidney beans, plus a variety called Calypso that were a crisp black and white in a perfect yin-yang pattern. There was even pasta made in Minneapolis from Minnesota flour; in fact, she said, it was for that very reason that her group had drawn their local limit at 250 miles.

I, on the other hand, could look forward to my homebound flight the next day, and then a winter salad of kale, anise, and mizuna. "Freshies!" said Sunny with obvious envy. She would wait for the first shoots of wild leek in May.

Though the light was dimming, we drove onto the backroads to pick Labrador tea in the forest. The air was crisp and fresh, without wind. Sunny explained to me how to give thanks to the plant, and to sprinkle a little American Spirit tobacco on the ground before I began. I could not bring myself to speak aloud, but I said thank you in my head, and meant it. To walk beneath the trees, silently following the trail of leaves poking up from the blue snow of twilight, was a gift. I recalled Sunny's careful log of her household food costs over the year so far. She clocked in at sixty-six dollars a week. "That's the same as the budget you get on welfare," Sunny said proudly; the federal food-stamp ceiling is $278 per two-person household each month. Sunny doesn't need any help from the government—she eats like a queen, if the queen of an unusual kingdom—but it seems that farmers do. The state of Minnesota offers special instructions for farming families who need to apply for food stamps, assuring them that their land will not count against them as an asset. The ultimate irony of modern agriculture—full fields and empty stomachs.

For my farewell breakfast, Sunny made pancakes with acorn flour she had ground herself. She laid out local maple syrup and butter she had churned. Finally, she mixed us each a drink: wild highbush cranberry juice with an elixir of violets and honey. How many violets had it taken to make that little jar of sweetness? "Hundreds," she said, and I marveled at the reminder of summer abundance.

Heaven in a glass. That was Minnesota. And what is Vancouver? Raw oysters on the half shell and a goblet of white wine. Life would be dreary without its luxuries, and to find them in their place, in their season, was to experience the world as a treasure house.

So this is the end of the world, I thought. Funny how it only seemed like a beginning.

—

Home from midwinter Minnesota, I managed to get James on the phone. He was on an assignment in Malawi, thirty hours away by plane. It is one of the poorest countries in Africa, and he sounded drained, more so through the hollow crackling of an international cell phone.

"I ate ants," he said. "They were actually pretty good. Like beer nuts. And did you know you can eat bean leaves?"

"Just how poor are people there? I mean, do bean leaves actually taste good?" I asked.

"Well, pretty good."

"This from a man who eats ants."

"I did try something that I didn't like. *Thelele.* Some kind of okra leaf. It tastes fine, but the texture is exactly—*exactly*—like mucus."

Many people spend the night before an overseas trip leaning across a bar with their friends. James made cheese. He and Ruben spent hours in the procedure, which at one point involved using their arms, submerged to the armpits, to stir a huge cauldron. Ruben had found a website with step-by-step instructions and photos, the closest the internet comes to learning the art at the elbow of an aging relative. It was not living, breathing community, but it was a reasonable facsimile. Olive and I drank wine, occasionally checking in on the revealed mysteries of curds and whey, and cottage cheese, and finally Ruben's cheese press of tin cans, old milk crates, and bicycle tubes.

"You're in a different world now, I guess," I said into the phone.

Yes and no, he seemed to say. As we spoke, 4 million people in Malawi were facing a famine. It was bizarre, said James, to see a country going hungry with every inch of earth seemingly cov-

ered with lush fields. Last year's harvest, hurt by drought, was
nearly used up, and the new crops had yet to ripen. But famine
is rarely as simple as a shortage of food. In Malawi's case, the
causes ranged widely, from the social disruption of epidemic
AIDS, to climate change, to corruption, to the chaotic policy demands of international lenders and donor nations. There is the
fact that Malawi's farmers must compete with the world's wealth-
iest; as Nicholas Stern, chief economist of the World Bank,
noted in 2002, every day the average European cow receives
$2.50 in subsidies while 75 percent of Africans get by on less
than two dollars. But there is also the question of the food itself.
Much of Malawi, which is not quite as large as Pennsylvania,
was cleared for tobacco fields during nearly seventy-five years as
a British protectorate. Corn was heavily adopted as a food crop,
though it is fickle in Malawian soil and many farmers now de-
pend on Central and South America's traditional "three sisters"
planting technique—growing squash, beans, and corn together.
It is a frail food system, almost totally dislocated from the ecology of its place. Not surprisingly, the U.S. National Research
Council has recently begun to advocate a return to African
vegetable and fruit crops as "powerful tools" for tackling hunger,
malnutrition, and poverty. James had noted that one traditional
cure for *njala*—the deadly weakening from hunger, or, in recent
years, AIDS—is a bundle of local plant medicines served in a
bowl of native cowpeas.

Two sets of photos had arrived by e-mail, James said. The first
came from his brother David, and showed David's son, Keir, taking his very first steps. The second set, taken with almost as
much tenderness, was from Ruben. It showed two blocks of

cheese. Because he and James were first-time cheese makers and still half-certain that the process would go perilously wrong, Ruben had stamped each wax-dipped round with a skull and crossbones. Death's-head cheese.

I laughed. "Don't you wish you were here?"

When at last we were together again, it was in Mérida, the cultural capital of the Yucatán Peninsula, in Mexico. February had been one of the craziest months of our lives. Minnesota, Malawi, Mexico.

I'm not sure what made us choose the almost literal hole-in-the-wall with the plastic chairs and fluorescent lights and soccer on mute in the corner. I believe we heard laughter, and I convinced myself there was something special about the place. James teased me for my unshakable belief that every greasy spoon we might walk into would be the one with the world's best homemade pie and real whipped cream. Yes, I was forever disappointing myself. But here we were in Mexico, and here was a real mariachi plucking music beautiful enough to make you want to cry, and in fact some of the Mexicans were doing just that. My faith in the world was justified. There was not a single touristic flourish in sight; the guitar player was simply making music for his friends. No sombreros or margaritas or sequins, just dusty jeans and button-up shirts askew at the end of a beery afternoon, and when the mariachi stopped playing, a magician took over. The magician—he was a master of gesture. He made a coin vanish in his hand, and then slyly produced it from behind James's ear. It was only when the man at the next table drew his finger meaningfully across his mouth that I understood the magician was mute.

But who needed chatter? We had *sopa de lima,* lime soup. Superb lime soup, simmered so long that the green rinds were soft. A single sense, taste, was all we needed. The ingredients— chicken broth, tomatoes, limes, green chilies—were fresh and undoubtedly local, the simple secret of the soup's rich flavor.

We had come to Mexico for the wedding of our friends Nils and Tammy, from Toronto. An oddity of life in a country as vast as Canada is that it often costs no more to bring scattered friends and family together in a destination like Mexico or Hawaii, served by inexpensive charter flights, than in the place that you live. And so we descended on Isla Mujeres, leaving behind February slush for a beach house shared with friends. The island had once been home to a Mayan fortress, and is now the more human-scale partner to the beachfront skyscrapers across the bay in Cancún. It would be a week of sunburn and piña coladas, but we no longer felt any need to leave our 100-mile diet behind. Wherever we went, well, that's the place we would be. Within twenty minutes of arriving, James had learned from a taxi driver that the island's signature dish, dating back perhaps three millennia to Mayan times, was barbecued fish *tikinxic* (pronounced *teek-een-SHEEK*).

Which is how we ended up beneath the tin roof of a cook's shack on Los Lancheros beach at the self-proclaimed "house of tikinxic." The chef was a man of few words who had been baked from the top down by the sun and from the bottom up by his long cooking pit.

"Fresh fish. The freshest!" he said, when James asked in Spanish the key ingredient to a good tikinxic.

"But what gives it the red color?"

The man reached for what appeared to be a bucket of house paint, complete with a brush. *"Achiote,"* he said, describing a ruddy seed that is ground into paste. He made a motion to show how he cuts a fish in half through its back, the butterfly filleting style. "Salt the fish—a lot of salt. Then mix the achiote with lime juice. You apply it like this." He pantomimed painting the red sauce onto the fish.

"Is it spicy?"

"Not spicy!" he shot back, turning to his grill. "Tikinxic should not bite!"

All of which seemed simple enough, until we mentioned our interest in cooking a tikinxic to anybody else. We were told to buy two balls of achiote paste, or four, or eight. To mix them with lime juice, or water, or a little cooking oil. We were advised to add one bulb of garlic—or that garlic must not be added. Grouper was the fish to use, except that snapper was the only acceptable choice.

In the end, we listened to whoever had the ingredients for sale. The real *lancheros,* the boatmen of the local fishing cooperative, sold us four silver torpedoes of *coronado* caught that morning. At the open-air market, an elderly woman weighed the fish in her hand and dropped eight balls of achiote into a bag. We bought limes and garlic, a sack of charcoal, and, at the next stall, 2 pounds of still-warm tortillas for a dollar.

A few hours after dark we had a platter heaped with fish, its flesh bright red and smoky, with the delicate tartness of achiote.

We ate it with *bayo* beans and tortillas and pineapple salsa and chalky local cheese, and ten good friends walked away from the table fed and happy on a 100-mile meal.

To really understand Yucatecan cuisine, though, we had to go to Mérida, the capital city of the peninsula. This was the advice of Eduardo Seijo Solís, the operator of the region's pioneering gastronomical tour. Though Mérida is a beautiful colonial capital with one of the oldest remaining churches in the New World, it has no beaches and no visible Mayan ruins. Few tourists can be bothered with the three-hour drive from Cancún. Along the way, we wondered how the Yucatán had any cuisine at all. The asphalt of the modern toll highway beelined through twin walls of brambles that sprouted from the pits of a limestone moonscape.

"There are a lot of rocks in the soil here," Seijo had acknowledged over the phone. "In fact, there is very little soil."

Yucatecan ingredients are a roll call of plants and animals that can survive the difficult conditions, drawn from Mayan, Spanish, and Caribbean influences. Number one on the list, though, had roots in Indonesia: the habanero pepper. "Some people think it comes from Havana, but this is not true," said Seijo. "It came with the Spanish from the island of Java. But in the whole Spanish dominion, from here south to Tierra del Fuego, the habanero stayed only in the Yucatán and became part of our cuisine. The habaneros grown here are the spiciest in the world." Seijo's revelations suggested that local eating was far from stagnant, dull, or provincial. Waves of change through trade and war have always swept over the world. People tested which seeds would take root in their native soil, and the new foods became the authentic tastes of home.

To find the habanero or any other delicacy in Mérida, we followed the decorous streets of the sixteenth-century colonial center into the chaos of the Lucas de Gálvez Market. We were overwhelmed by odors of shellfish and offal, but the stall run by Eduardo Quetzal was fragrant. He was a spice merchant. We had sought him out for *relleno negro,* a mysterious, inky paste that we had sampled the night before at Los Almendros Restaurant, an institution in Yucatecan cuisine.

"It's a chili—and *only* a chili," said Quetzal, a stone-faced man whose voice revealed kindness. "They're burnt to ash over coals and then ground up." A family-sized serving might require *4 pounds* of dried peppers, and yet the sauce's heat is released as a low, slow burn. James was a fan, but I couldn't decide whether I liked it or not; the flavor had a hint of kerosene, and its pure blackness was alarming as a sauce. This I can say: it was exciting to find something so unlike anything else I'd eaten, anywhere on Earth.

"How much of this food would come from one hundred miles away or less?" asked James.

"Almost all of it," said Quetzal, casting an eye to the neat stacks of seasonal radishes, squash, *chaya* spinach, corn, potatoes, habaneros. Then he began a list of impossible names: Yaxcopoil, Oxkutzcab, Xcanatún. "Go out to the villages if you want to see where the food comes from," he said. "Go out and meet the Maya."

And so we did. Along nearly empty backroads, we sampled a liquor made from a cactus that can also be used to make rope. We shared pit-roasted corn with three women who embroidered the traditional Mayan *huipil* blouses. In the "Mayan Andes" we tasted the milky succulence of the purple *caimito* fruit. We enjoyed a re-freshment sold by women at roadside stalls: sour oranges cut in half and dusted with hand-ground chili powder. In a hotel kitch-enette near Playa del Carmen, we cooked eggs in a pumpkin-seed sauce. Not once did we need to eat food from beyond a 100-mile boundary. In many places, a 10-mile limit would have been enough.

Most of the world still eats this way. In the current age of globalization, the standout defender of the right to feed oneself from the place one lives is La Via Campesina, an international movement of peasant organizations. Among their priorities is a demand that food be removed from the deregulation agenda of the World Trade Organization.

The issue is much more than a difference in philosophy. In India, for example, 17,107 farmers committed suicide in 2003, the most recent year for which figures were available. Most had been unable to feed themselves and their families after losing government protection from competing agroindustrial imports and taking on crippling debt to purchase the pesticides, chemi-cal fertilizers, and genetically modified seeds needed to "mod-ernize" their farms. Mexico is another place that has borne the brunt of agricultural globalization. Since a free-trade deal with the United States and Canada came into effect on New Year's Day 1994—a date marked by the emergence of a guerrilla army of masked rebels, the Zapatistas—a glut of subsidized corn from America has overwhelmed Mexico's two million small farmers, for whom corn is a traditional staple. Many have lost their liveli-hoods; dwindling alongside them was the diversity of Mexico's 5,000 varieties of maize.

It is still possible, though, to taste the living history. James and I ended our Yucatán wanderings at Chichén Itzá, the 1,400-year-old ruins of a Mayan city. Our guide, a local named José Cob, pointed out the Temple of the Three Lintels, the Group of the Thousand Columns, the House of the Deer. Just past the stepped Pyramid of Kukulcán, he called a few words of Mayan to some friends on a break from work. We asked what was in the large pot an old man carried.

"You want to try it?" said Cob, doubtful but a little pleased. "This," he said, "is what my father and I used to take with us into the jungle when he worked as a woodcutter." The elderly vendor handed us a serving of *pozole* to share. It was a ritual as much as a meal. A pinch of salt. A mouthful of warm hominy mash from a dried gourd. And a bite of raw habanero. It was a whole and simple meal, drawn from earth that has been worked by the Maya since Chichén Itzá was still on the drawing board.

A few minutes later we passed one more Mayan-style edifice, which appeared to be the most popular stop on the ancient site. The concession stand. "And that," said Cob, "is the Temple of Coca-Cola."

It was raining. We were home.

The taxi pulled away and I felt the first cold drops against my face. We had passed on the meager airline lunch, choosing instead to fast in anticipation of what felt, now, like the only real food.

"What will we have for lunch?" I asked.

"Potatoes?" James said, and we laughed.

The door to our apartment jammed against the pile of junk

mail stuffed through the slot while we'd been away. On top was a card from our newly married friend Nils, posted from Toronto and addressed to the "50-Meter Diet Club":

Tam and I have been living off of spiders, flies, bees, and dust mites since we returned to the Big Smoke—we feel as thin as runway models! Have set up pigeon traps on the balcony but have only been able to catch hummingbirds . . .

I stepped over the heap and pushed my way in with my baggage. Bumping into the bedroom, I froze. The cupboard. The door was open a crack on the potato cupboard.

"We didn't close the potato cupboard," I said with genuine shock. "The light will have ruined them. They'll be green."

James slipped in beside me, dropped his pack, and put his hands on his hips. "I'm sure we did close it," he said. A creepy tone entered his voice. "Maybe *they* opened it. Maybe they pushed it open *with their eyes.*"

We looked at each other with raised eyebrows. James lifted his foot, toed the cupboard door wide open. Inside was a lunatic, pale pink tangle of sprouted eyes, some nearly two feet long and each roaming in search of light and earth. The potatoes really had tried to make their escape. "Look at those," I said. "They're growing little leaf buds." It was true. The potatoes themselves looked like nearly empty sacks, but the tips of the long, white antlers were flecked with green. All they wanted was to grow, to be reborn with the approaching season. "It's almost spring," I said. "We only have three weeks to go." I felt wistful, but James's laughter was contagious.

The winter was taking its toll. The pickles had lost crispness, and a small squash had imploded into a powder-dry husk. Nonetheless, we had an incredible surplus of good food; the freezer and cupboards were more than half full. We still had a sturdy blue-green Hubbard squash, the size of a strongman's medicine ball. For the next three weeks, we'd be feasting.

James made lunch: wild rice and lentils from Minnesota, a still-moist old beet, walnuts, a white sauce with Yucatán chilies, dill, onions, garlic, and the usual Oregon salt. He also boiled a potato, first trimming off the eyes. Knowing he would only ignore my warnings, I turned on the radio and stretched out on the couch. I would leave him to his experiment.

"You know what these potatoes taste like?" he called out.

"What?"

"They taste like the potatoes you get in restaurants."

I was distracted by a change in the room, which I couldn't quite place. I leaned up on my elbows and looked outside. The clouds had broken. Soon the radio murmured an alarm—there were traffic jams everywhere. Cars were crawling through the streets like fearful animals. Why? It was sunny. The low sun glared on the wet world and blinded the city; no one had carried sunglasses for months. But for once no one was angry at the delay. No horns blared. The moment hinted at grand transformations: winter to spring; chill darkness to warmth; life moving forward though the end of the road was obscured by sudden light.

EPILOGUE

IT IS NO LESS DIFFICULT TO WRITE SENTENCES IN A RECIPE
THAN SENTENCES IN <u>MOBY-DICK</u>.

ANNIE DILLARD

The final day of our 100-mile diet came early. For years, March 21 had been the traditional first day of spring. In 2006, it changed. The astronomers and calendar makers consulted their charts and declared that the vernal equinox now arrived a full day sooner. The morning of March 20 dawned with winter's same old pabulum sky, but our year of eating locally was over. We could eat anything, anything on Earth. Alisa climbed into the bath.

"What do you want for breakfast?" called out James from the kitchen. "You want to go to Solly's? Get a big bagel with lox and a cinnamon bun?" Splooshing noises came from the bathroom. A long silence. "Or just potatoes and eggs?"

"Potatoes and eggs seem fine to me," said Alisa.

Well: another local meal. We had brought the adventure to a close the night before with a blowout feast. Keri and Ron were there, the couple who had come for the very first 100-mile dinner, and so were Ruben and Olive, who had become so much a part of the experiment. The table was heavy with the usual cornucopia. Though we were down to our last jar of tomatoes, the new year had been mild enough that we could serve a salad of winter greens. The highlight, however, was the ceremonial cutting of the round of death's-head cheese that had aged in our cupboard for six weeks. James and Ruben each placed their hands on the handle of the knife, like a couple posing with a wedding cake. Then they cleaved the block in half.

"It looks cheesy," Keri offered.

Ruben held a chunk to his nose. "Smells like cheese," he declared.

There was reluctance in the room. A few days earlier a group of us had sampled the block of cheese that had been stored at Ruben's house, but then, his had matured in the fridge. James had aged his death's-head at room temperature, and some worrisome yellow liquid had wept out of the rind. It looked and smelled like cheese, but then, anaerobic toxins have no odor, and no taste.

"I think I'm going to go jump off the balcony," said Keri casually, but Ruben headed her off with a slice from the block. Everyone took a piece. James took the first bite and seemed pleasantly surprised.

"It's salty," he said.

"Salty like sausage?" asked Keri.

"No," said James, as the rest of the table sampled their slices. "Salty like road salt."

"It tastes like salty cheese . . . with salt on it," said Ron, and the laughter cut the tension.

Around the dinner table the wine and the conversation flowed.

We solved most of the world's problems, recounted old stories, composed a list of all the ridiculous things that had turned
people—other people—into millionaires, such as plastic bris-
tles for whisk brooms in China. A dictionary was hauled out to
differentiate *antimony,* which is a semimetallic element, from *antimony,* which is a contradiction between two reasonable beliefs.
At last Keri, who was sober, asked the unavoidable question:
"What are you going to eat tomorrow?"

"Count Chocula for breakfast," said James with a straight
face. "Pizza Pops for lunch. I don't know what for dinner. Maybe
a McCain Deep and Delicious?"

"With cheese baked into the crust!" said Ruben.

"Isn't a McCain Deep and Delicious a chocolate cake?" Olive
asked. There were murmurs of agreement.

Ron nearly climbed from his chair. "How about a McCain
Deep and Delicious chocolate cake," he said, *"with cheese baked
into the crust?"*

"It's like listening to insane people," said Keri, almost to
herself.

Alisa came to the table with the final course, a plate of homemade crackers with cheese. The death's-head variety had been
quietly set aside, replaced by local Camembert, brie, and a blend
of Derby and Asiago.

"We've never made crackers," Keri said thoughtfully. She
takes pride in being one of the few of our generation who still
produces home preserves.

"Have you made cheese?" Ruben demanded.

"No."

"Pasta?"

"No."

"Yogurt?"

"Yes."

"Soap?" Ruben barked.

"No."

"Then what do you keep him around for?" Ruben asked Keri, thumbing over his shoulder at Ron.

Six months have passed. It is a rare cloudless day on the west coast of Vancouver Island, the Graveyard of the Pacific, and we are rowing for the open ocean. James has his hands on the oars and his back to the bow. Alisa is in the stern, and might be mistaken for some Victorian lady out on the Thames with her beau except that she points silently now and again to direct James, who can't see where he's going. That, and the fact that there are bald eagles everywhere.

It takes twelve hours to get here from Vancouver. By car, by ferry across the Salish Sea, then car again, then four hours on the outport steamer *Frances Barkley*. Its last stop is Bamfield, population 300 and the most remote village still inside the 100-mile circle that had fed us for a year. Here, brightly colored starfish rest in the clear water, and purple anemones like pompoms cling to the docks. A fresh tang of salt hangs in the air.

We can't ignore the irony, all these hours of travel in the name of local eating, but it is, for us, a necessary journey. What we are about to do is, above all else, symbolic. We have attempted to reinvent our way of eating. Is it still possible, in a global age, in an age of fast food, to live off the land that surrounds us? It is. In the end there was only a single, nagging foodstuff in the cupboards that was not a part of the place we call home.

Salt.

The little rowboat noses into the countering wind. At least we are going in the right direction now. We had started out down a dead-end channel that turned out to be a natural receptacle for an inflowing tide of marine oil, garbage, and sewage from Bamfield. More than an hour at the oars brought us back against the current to the mouth of the inlet. Just a few more yards to round Aguilar Point.

And then—nothing. A blue horizon, forever and ever to Japan. The open Pacific Ocean rushing in as clear and clean as the air. James keeps the boat steady against the tide, and Alisa dips a jug and begins to fill a huge stainless steel pot with salt water.

Human beings do not need salt in its stand-alone crystalline form—it is not a true necessity. According to anthropologists and archaeologists, many hunter-gatherer societies did not make or trade salt, but acquired enough to survive through the content of their wild foods. It would never have occurred to the original peoples of the Pacific Northwest, with their diet of seafood and kelp, to make salt. Yet the seasoning has become a pillar of civilization, so much so that most modern people consume far more than is healthy. The salt industry cites 14,000 uses—from extinguishing oil fires to relieving tired feet—without even including blood, sweat, and tears. Salt is a critical ingredient for curing, smoking, pickling, and fermenting. It is helpful to the cheesemaking process, though it is best to apply it sparingly.

The recorded history of saltmaking stretches back 2,800 years to China. By the time the technique was written down it was already ancient, and it is more or less that same process which we now brought to Bamfield: fill an urn with seawater, boil off the water, and collect the salt crystals that are left behind. Other parts of the world, such as northern Africa, have saline lakes that act as natural saltworks, and many of Europe's cities—consider Salzburg—were founded alongside salt wells or mines. Boiling down brine, though, has never faded as a way to make salt.

Few people think of salt as a product with a place of origin. Salt comes out of a box. But everything comes from somewhere, and now there are gourmet salts from Hawaii, New Zealand, Egypt, the Himalayas. On the southern shore of the Algarve in Portugal, artisan saltmakers skim fleeting shavings off the liquid surface of salt pans—the *fleur de sel,* now a staple of luxury restaurants. They do the same in the French salt marshes of the Guérande peninsula. The process can be made elaborate, but on the other hand, oceans cover some 70 percent of the surface of the Earth. Salt is everywhere. When there is nothing else, a person might always make salt.

In 1815 the British government, then in control of India, famously banned the production of salt in that country by anyone but the imperial crown; even gathering salt for one's own purposes was a punishable offense. Rebellion followed, but by 1863 the people of India could choose to buy salt imported from Britain, or not to buy salt at all. More than sixty years later, the viceroy of England received a letter stating that Britain's colonial presence was about to be challenged, and "the beginning will be made with this evil"—the salt laws. It was signed by an emerging leader of India's independence movement, Mahatma Gandhi, who was born in Porbandar, a town near the vast salt marsh called the Rann of Kutch.

On March 12, 1930, Gandhi and seventy-eight men from his ashram set out on foot for a 240-mile journey to the sea. Twenty-three days later they arrived at the salt flats with thousands of supporters and the eyes of the world on a sixty-year-old barefoot guru who had not eaten salt himself for six years. He led prayers all night and, at first light, purified himself in the Indian Ocean. Then he walked up the beach, broke off a crust from the salt marsh, and proceeded to boil it into pure salt.

Our 100-mile diet hadn't ended, not really. The day after the final dinner, at lunchtime, James used a dash of black pepper on some leftover pasta. Alisa suggested a nice Indian place for dinner, and we ordered jackfruit, which probably came from Southeast Asia or Brazil. A few favorites have slowly made their way back into the kitchen—lemons, and rice, and beer. Many others, like bland bananas and white sugar, haven't yet. For us, the balance of global versus local food has been reversed. It comes down to this: we just like the new way better.

It's been easier the second time through the seasons. The asparagus harvest was a success, though the berries came late and the farmers' markets were delayed by a cool spring. Steve Johansen brought in the spot prawns, and this year the sockeye salmon came back to the Fraser in the millions, ringing every bell on the *Black Heart*'s trolling lines. Nature, as unpredictable as ever. We still had the pleasure of new discoveries: an old-fashioned red carrot, far better in stews than the orange ones; almonds from Victoria; side-stripe shrimp from the Pacific shore. Alisa met a woman who had seen with her own eyes a mature olive tree in East Vancouver. James grew tomatillos in the garden. We canned the tomatoes side by side.

We did not buy real estate, but in June, after eleven weeks of training, Alisa fulfilled a dream: she rode a century, the cycling equivalent of a marathon. Her route took her past Fraser Valley farms, across the border to Washington's Whatcom County, halfway up the volcanic cone of Mount Baker, and back again; James followed in the little red car, doling out home-baked granola bars. At the finish line, Alisa grinned and crunched a piece of kelp to replace her lost salts. A century, of course, is a ride of exactly 100 miles.

And the idea continued to germinate. Local-eating experiments were launched from Britain to Australia; from Albany, New York, to Eugene, Oregon. Sunny Johnson from Minnesota was stuck with engine problems in Utah on the day that her own year of local eating ended. She ate a Subway sandwich at the highway's edge—but she was headed west to Los Angeles to pitch a television program about foraging wild plants. Just north of Vancouver, a fellow named Chris Hergesheimer sowed an everyman-size patch of soil with spring wheat and blogged his crop's progress from seed to baked bread. We asked a Vancouver Island farmer to plant black and pinto beans, as well as chickpeas, for local eaters, but the crop couldn't keep ahead of the weeds. A scientist in Antarctica wrote to report that his research station kept a greenhouse, and as the first days of autumn once again approached, Alisa's youngest sister made jam for the first time in her life, from blackberries picked in her mother's backyard.

Then came news from the town of Powell River, not far north of Vancouver but accessible only by ferry. A group had come together. They would attempt to sign up fifty people to eat from within 50 miles for five weeks. In the end, more than 250 people chose to participate, as well as restaurants, grocers, a butcher, and the fish shop. Powell River, population 13,000, is a mill town of declining fortunes—another castaway of the global economic juggernaut. "Hardly any of our local farmers make a living off their farms," said Lyn Adamson, one of the key organizers of the Powell River project. "We're hoping that if they feel enough consumer confidence they'll grow more—or people will feel confident enough to start new farms."

Every nook and cranny of the cottage we have rented in Bamfield is musty with steam. We have made our own pilgrimage to the sea. The world is not watching, though a curious tomcat is. We've left the doors open to the morning sun and the sounds of the port: outboard motors, mewing gulls, a sea lion clearing its throat. It is less than 50 paces to the ocean shore.

There is nothing miraculous about making salt. Put the seawater on the stove and boil it down. When the water is nearly gone, set small batches to simmer in a frying pan. Then wait. One minute the liquid is bubbling, and the next, the thinnest imaginable crystals have formed on the surface. The *fleur de sel.*

Actually, there is something miraculous about making salt.

The sun is high again on the ragged edge of British Columbia.

Alisa walks into the kitchen. "Hey," she says softly. The last of the seawater is turning to steam. James appears at her shoulder. He takes hold of the pan and tilts it, and with a wooden scraper Alisa carries the damp crystals to a waiting bowl. It is already nearly full. The salt is a dazzling white pile, enough to last through another year.

ACKNOWLEDGMENTS

Books begin with a leap of faith. Ours started with editor David Beers of the TheTyee.ca, and with Anne McDermid and Emma Parry, who saw the book in our online column before we did. Publishing is a collective act, and many more thanks are due, not least to Shaye Areheart and John Glusman, who took to our idea with gusto, and to Anne Collins, an able wordsmith and a farm gal to boot. Many who offered aid, advice, and sometimes a bed along the way went unnamed in these pages; they include Mike Norrie, George Laundry, Usha Rautenbach, Briony Penn, Mike Doehnel, Terry Glavin, Kirk Safford, and Michael Ableman. James reserves special thanks for farmer Dieter Eisenhawer of Metchosin. The authors of the *Good Housekeeping Cook Book,* 1944 edition, also deserve to be named: Katharine Fisher and Dorothy B. Marsh. Parents, grandparents, elders—thank you.

Founding 100milediet.org was a surprisingly complex task. Biro Creative supplied valuable ideas and helped turn them into reality. Other key supporters were Joel Solomon and the Endswell Foundation, Farm Folk/City Folk, Capers Community

ACKNOWLEDGMENTS

Markets, Small Potatoes Urban Delivery, and the National Farmers Union. Denise McCabe, Vanessa Richmond, Kelly Kuryk, Shirlene Cote, and Jeff Nield have been valuable allies, as have Lyn Adamson and Kathie Mack, the catalysts behind the outstanding Powell River local eating project. Hats off, too, to Andrea Carlson, Sue Alexander, and Raincity Grill. Last but not least, a debt of gratitude to the many people who have written to share their own local eating stories and recipes.

As we worked on this book, we became aware of the emerging local foods movement. Several leaders warrant recognition: Sage Van Wing and the Locavores (locavores.com); Jennifer Maiser and the Eat Local Challenge (eatlocalchallenge.com); Local Harvest (localharvest.org); Treehugger.com; Slow Food; and Gary Paul Nabhan, author of *Coming Home to Eat.* Countless others— too many to name—are promoting a saner food system, the protection of agricultural land, and a better deal for farmers. This fact gives us much hope.

While this book is at heart a memoir, we did our utmost to support every statement of fact with authoritative and primary sources. Several excellent background sources will be of interest to many readers: Christopher D. Cook's *Diet for a Dead Planet;* Alan Davidson's *The Oxford Companion to Food;* Terry Glavin's *Waiting for the Macaws;* John Gowdy's *Limited Wants, Unlimited Means;* Brian Halweil's *Eat Here;* Deborah Madison's *Local Flavors;* Marion Nestle's *Food Politics;* Michael Pollan's *The Omnivore's Dilemma;* and Eric Schlosser's *Fast Food Nation.* We cannot sign off without recognizing public libraries and archives— essential institutions that deserve and require our support. Finally, a toast to the writers in the Vancouver FCC, who are perpetual inspirations: Deborah Campbell, Charles Montgomery, Brian Payton, Chris Tenove, and John Vaillant. To whomever we've forgotten, we hope to be forgiven.